LISTEN TO YOUR BODY

Listen to Your Body

The Wisdom of the Dao

BISONG GUO AND ANDREW POWELL

A Latitude 20 Book

University of Hawai'i Press
Honolulu

ı

14 13 12 11 10 09   8 7 6 5 4 3

Library of Congress Cataloging-in-Publication Data
Guo, Bisong.
  Listen to your body : the wisdom of the Dao / Bisong Guo and Andrew Powell.
    p.   cm.
  "A Latitude 20 book."
  ISBN 978-0-8248-2381-8 (alk. paper)
  ISBN 978-0-8248-2466-2 (pbk. : alk. paper)
  1. Hygiene, Taoist.   I. Title: Wisdom of the Dao.   II. Powell, Andrew.
  III. Title

RA781 .G86 2001
613'.0951—dc21

                                        2001027358

Excerpts from the *Tao Te Ching (Daodejing)* are taken from the translation by Gia-Fu Feng and Jane English (Wildwood House, 1973; Reprint, 1986).

Designed by inari information services, inc.

Printed by The Maple-Vail Book Manufacturing Group

Contents

Foreword   ix
Acknowledgments   xiii
Introduction   xv

PART ONE
The Miracle of the Human Body

The Cosmos as a Living Organism   3
Yin and *Yang*: Nature's Energy Balance   11
The Meridians   15
The Flow of Q*i* in Nature   24
Harnessing Nature's Q*i*: The Three *Dantian*   27

PART TWO
The Information System of the Body

The Natural Human Life Span   33
Recognizing the Signals Your Body Sends   36
Case Studies from a Specialist Clinic   42
      The Body's Warning Signals Ignored   42
      Live Now, Pay Later   43
      The Ring that Changed a Woman's Life   45
      The Engineer Who Ran out of Steam   47

"Doctor, What's Wrong with Me?"   49
A Hysterectomy Avoided   51
Joints Cracking—*Yin* Lacking!   52
What the Back Can Tell Us about Q*i*   53
The TCM Approach to Multiple Sclerosis   56
A Child with Asthma: No Need for Steroids   59
Who Is the Patient, Mother or Baby?   61
Holiday Syndromes   63

PART THREE
Learning to Trust the Wisdom of Your Body

Mind and Body in Harmony   69
Relaxed Mind, Relaxed Body   71
Ancient Medicine: A Hundred Generations of Study   75
The Art of Knowing Your Q*i*   79
    Whole Body Reactions   81
    Specific Body Reactions   82
    Assessing the State of Your Health   83
    Protecting Your Q*i*   88

PART FOUR
The Daily Care of Your Body

The Biorhythms of *Yin* and *Yang*   93
The Right Way to Start the Day   97
The Art of Breathing   99
The Rhythm of the Four Seasons   104
Water as Medicine   107
Washing Is a Skill!   114
How to Dress   120
Eating Wisely, Eating Well   124
Natural Body Functions   130
Medicinal Plants   132
Drinking Alcohol: Vice or Virtue?   136
Q*i* and Sex   139

Traveling with Ease   145
Keeping Your Home from Harm   150
Preparing for Sleep   151
Enjoy Aging with the Help of Your Qi   155

Postscript   159
Index   163

Foreword

YESTERDAY I returned to work after a short break. "How are you?" a colleague asked. "I'm well, thank you," I replied, a simple, familiar form of greeting posed and responded to quickly and automatically. But how was I really? A few aches and pains perhaps, but that's normal enough, isn't it? Apprehensive about the day ahead maybe, but that's how work is, isn't it? It could be that any number of things were not quite right within me, but did I know? This book asks us to enter the place between that question and answer, to make a space between the two, and to listen to what our bodies are telling us. Externally the greeting and response may remain the same, but internally we have the opportunity to hear and respond to the messages our body is giving us and to enjoy more fully both our health and ourselves.

In this book, Dr. Guo and Dr. Powell have managed to capture and communicate the essence of the Daoist philosophy of health in a way that is both challenging and informative. Between them, the authors can count many years of clinical experience and much expertise in Traditional Chinese Medicine and western medicine. This unique combination enables them to offer the reader access to insight and knowledge previously unavailable. They have been able to synthesize and interpret ancient wisdom using case studies and illustrations with clarity and acuity. These days we are bombarded with recipes for health, so-called orthodox and alternative. Yet all too often, the scientific evidence seemingly confirms and then contradicts its own conclusions. It is indeed a confusing world! If, however, we are willing to stop compartmentalizing our lives and begin to recognize that health (in all its states) is part of our "being in the world," then the simple messages of this text are likely to have a profound effect.

There is increasing recognition among scholars and scientists that in order to promote health and recovery, complex interactions between a condition and its treatment must be taken into account. In rehabilitation following stroke, for example, it has been shown that although acute intervention is needed during the first twenty-four to forty-eight hours to enable the body's systems to stabilize, it is the physical, psychological, and social treatment that follows which promotes recovery. The promotion of health and the rehabilitation of the individual with poor health are part of a multidimensional process. As such, there is no quick fix, and there has to be impact and maintenance in all areas of life for effect to be demonstrated. In Parkinson's disease, for example, a condition for which there is no cure, recent research has indicated that life-enhancing strategies in which patient, caregiver, therapist, and doctor all take part, are most effective in enabling individuals to manage their impairments and disabilities. The net result of using such strategies (which maximize the individual's abilities across all daily functions) is to minimize the effect of the disease on everyday life.

This book illustrates a life-enhancing strategy based on the ancient and complex system of Traditional Chinese Medicine. This science differs from what we in the West, with our view of cause, effect, and controlled experimentation, have been taught. Nevertheless, western science has begun to scrutinize Daoist science and is increasingly finding evidence and explanations that should allow us to respect differences and share truths.

What, by the end of this book, will the reader have learned? This is no simplistic overview of Traditional Chinese Medicine. The authors have deliberately chosen to clear a path through what could have been a jungle of explanations by avoiding the temptation, as in many other texts, to present a theoretical treatise. Here we have exactly what we need to know and why we need to know it. By the end, we will have a template for managing the health of our own bodies, a daily plan, if you like. We will be familiar with how to listen to our own bodies and assess our energy or *qi*. Most importantly we will have an understanding of our biorhythms, day-to-day and month-to-month, and of the changing balance of *qi (yin and yang)* within our bodies. We will know how to balance and nurture both internal and environmental *qi* and how to protect and promote our health. We will have the opportunity to change not only ourselves but also our world, through the understanding that our bodies are inextricably intertwined physically and spiritually.

When we care for our bodies, we care for our spirit too, and caring for ourselves means also caring for the world we live in, since ultimately all are part of one whole. Daoist wisdom holds that it is not a question of mind over matter but of true harmony of body and mind. Then healing can take place.

We need to respond to this challenge, to take note and act with urgency if we are not to become complicit bystanders to our own demise. I have followed the guidance set out in *Listen to Your Body* for some months and can add that I believe we will learn from it what it feels like to be a good deal calmer and happier.

I commend to you these teachings as a strategy for life.

Dr. Rowena Plant
Professor of Rehabilitation/Therapy
University of Newcastle-upon-Tyne

Acknowledgments

THE AUTHORS wish to record their deep appreciation of the support and encouragement given by Colin McDermott, Liu Sola, Zhang Hongjing, and Hu Xiaoling in helping this book along its journey toward publication.

Introduction

WE ARE ALL living with our bodies twenty-four hours a day, every day of our lives. But how well do we know our bodies? Do we have to be doctors to understand what is going on? Do we need to hand over our bodies to a professional every time we get a symptom or rely on a prescription to put the problem right?

If you don't understand your body, seeing your doctor is the sensible thing to do. But the first step is working with the medicine that is right there in your own home—the natural medicine of the body. This book will help you use that natural medicine to maintain good health and to improve your condition if you already have a health problem.

Listen to Your Body deserves serious study. It offers a distillation of five thousand years of knowledge and brings the essence of that wisdom into our modern age for the benefit of all, young and old, well and infirm, patient and doctor. Here you will learn about the flow of energy within you that balances and maintains the health of every living cell. You will become aware of the rhythms that shape our lives. Such rhythms are found throughout nature: night follows day, the tides flow with the phases of the moon, the seasons come and go. All life on earth depends on these rhythms. If we listen to our bodies, we will soon detect the ebb and flow of many subtle changes that are going on all the time within us. But we won't notice them unless we pay careful attention, because so many activities of modern life are not geared to these biorhythms.

Listen to Your Body shows you how to tune in to the signals your body sends out that warn of a developing health problem. A variety of case histories are included to illustrate how theory and practice go together. Exercises and simple routines are given in detail. Prevention of illness and specific guidance for avoiding a number of common disorders are covered. All of this will help you to apply the natural medicine of the body to daily life. The result is a day-by-day program that promotes health, healing, and longevity.

The foundations of this book lie in the *Yijing* (or *I Ching*—The book of changes), whose origins are shrouded in antiquity, more than six thousand years ago. The *Yijing* was the first systematic account of the workings of the cosmos according to the principle of *yin* and *yang*. With the *Yijing* came the cultivation of the esoteric art of *qigong* and the development of Traditional Chinese Medicine. Archaelogical findings from the New Stone Age reveal that originally stone needles were used in the treatment of disease with acupuncture. Later, some four thousand years ago, the practice of applying burning herbs to the acupuncture points (now called moxibustion) was developed.

By the fifth century BC, in the Chunqiu Zhanguo period, stone needles had been supplanted by metal needles. This was a remarkable period. The framework of Traditional Chinese Medicine was now established, culminating in *The Yellow Emperor's Canon of Medicine*. The sage Laozi (Lao Tsu) summarized the spiritual essence of the Daoist way of life in the short but profound text of the *Daodejing (Dao De Ching)*, while in India Buddhism was taking root. Many centuries later, when Buddhism spread to China, a rich synthesis of Buddhism, the *Yijing*, Daoism, and Traditional Chinese Medicine took place that continues to the present day.

There have been a number of great sages in the Daoist tradition who have also been *qigong* masters, doctors of medicine, and experts in *fengshui*, and much of their sound advice is found in this book. The illustrious Wei Boyang, for example, who lived in the Han dynasty, wrote *Zhouyi cantongqi* (Kinship of the three and the book of changes), which describes the human body as a miniature cosmos, an understanding Wei Boyang reached through his integration of the *Yijing* with *qigong* and Daoist alchemical practice. Ge Hong, living in the Jin dynasty, gave detailed instructions on health care in *Baopuzi neipian* (Preservation-of-solidarity master). Sun Simiao, from the Tang dynasty, is honored for *Qianjinfang* (A thousand golden remedies). Later, in the Ming dynasty, books such as *Leixiuyaojue* (Collective aphorisms of *qigong* healthcare) brought together the teachings of many great masters on the law of the *Dao*, which means "the Way of Nature." Such books are still widely read in China.

The more visible aspect of the Daoist tradition, as in the art of *fengshui*, has readily caught the attention of the western mind. But for a real understanding of the *Dao*, the innermost principles of this wisdom need to be grasped. This is what the book sets out to do, with particular reference to health care, enabling the reader to take the necessary steps for long-lasting improvements in health, not superficially but from deep within. One condition is attached, however, and in fairness to the reader, it is given here at the start: change takes effort. As the Chinese saying goes, "Pancakes don't fall out of the sky!"

Modern society has profoundly alienated man from nature, and the cost to human health and happiness is only now beginning to be recognized. This book invites the reader to try a different approach to life, one that both listens to the workings of the human body and reaches out to the timeless majesty of the cosmos.

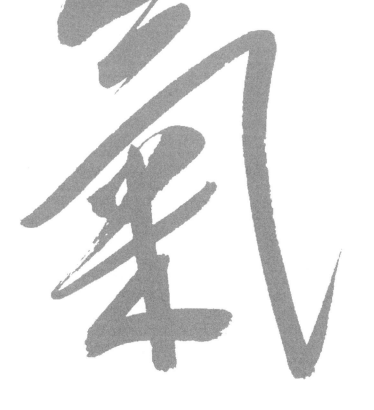

PART ONE

The Miracle of the Human Body

The Cosmos as a
Living Organism

The beginning of the universe
Is the mother of all things.
Knowing the mother, one also knows the sons.
Knowing the sons, yet remain in touch with the mother.

—Laozi, *Daodejing*

W **E USUALLY** think of our bodies as complete in themselves, separate from the air we breathe and the ground
we walk on. It is true that the body is a whole universe
in itself. But it is part and parcel of the total universe in which we live
and to which we are connected every minute of our lives.

When we look at a clear night sky, we see thousands of stars all
suspended in space in our own galaxy, and we know that our galaxy
is just one of millions reaching to infinity. Within our own bodies, we
too have galaxy upon galaxy. The energy of the stars we see outside
exists inside us, so that the internal space of the body is organized on
the same principles that govern the whole universe. (Imagine an
infinite set of Russian dolls, each one having a smaller, identical doll
inside it.) The galaxies all spin. Our own galaxy, the Milky Way, is
like a giant dinner plate spiraling round and round. Positioned near
its edge, our own solar system is itself revolving. Our planet also
spins around its geographic axis, having a geomagnetic field with a
north and south pole. The same magnetic force field is present in
every living cell, each with its positive and negative pole.

The human body as a whole similarly has its own force field. In China it is called *qi* (pronounced "chee"). *Qi* is made up of energy that is in constant motion, though mostly we are not paying attention to it. But *qi* is more than energy as we usually think of it.

Have you ever stopped to wonder how a galaxy keeps its shape? It isn't just a mass of stars haphazardly floating around in space. Rather, it is a gigantic system composed of millions of stars all moving together through the operation of the invisible force of gravity, which maintains its existence.

In the miniature universe of the human body, the unseen force that maintains us is the *qi*. It is a remarkable information system. It doesn't communicate in words, but we can learn how to read the messages it sends and find out what is going on inside us.

Qi possesses another striking characteristic: **Inside each part can be found a reflection of the whole.** Such structures are known as holograms. Scientists discovered how to create holograms in the 1960s when using coherent beams of light (lasers). Some scientists now describe the universe as a "holoverse."

To explain further, if you were to look at your face in a mirror that had a crack down the middle, you would normally expect to see half your face reflected back on each side of the crack. But in the case of a hologram, even if the mirror shattered, every piece, however small, would still contain a miniature reflection of your whole face.

The principle of the hologram lies at the heart of Traditional Chinese Medicine (TCM). Just as the cycle of the year contains 365 days, so within our body there are 365 acupuncture points. The calendar year has 12 months and our bodies have 12 major meridians, or energy channels. Within the body itself, the hand, foot, face, eye, and ear, for instance, all have maps of the whole body imprinted on them. Not only do these "living maps" allow us to get a picture of the whole body by looking at just one small part, such as the ear, but also inspecting the ear closely reveals what is wrong with the body as a whole. Thus treatment can be given to the whole body through the acupuncture points of the ear.

The tongue is also essential to diagnosis in TCM. Looking at the condition of the tongue is like turning on the television for the latest

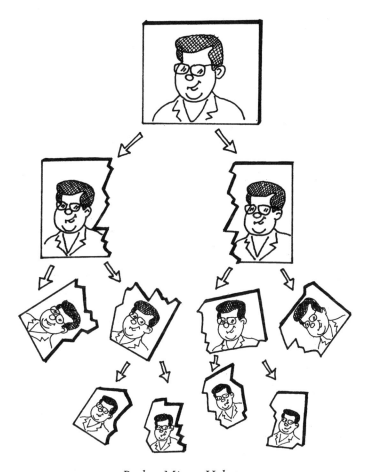

Broken Mirror Hologram

weather report. The color, size, coating, and presence of cracks all indicate very precisely the condition of the body. The tongue coating reflects the energy level and in good health shows a thin white coating. In fact, the tongue is a very sensitive organ and will look completely different after a successful acupuncture treatment. Even thoughts and emotions will change its appearance within seconds.

Think how rapidly the weather can change, from hour to hour and even from minute to minute. The wind, the clouds, the sun, and the temperature all combine to produce the climate surrounding us. Likewise, according to TCM, inside the body we have a climate of our own changing from minute to minute, with a balance of

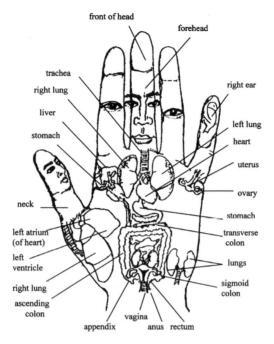

Left Palm

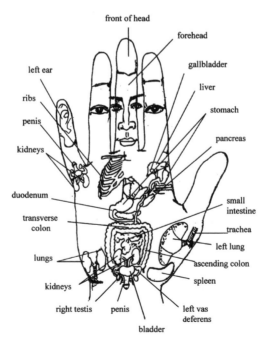

Right Palm

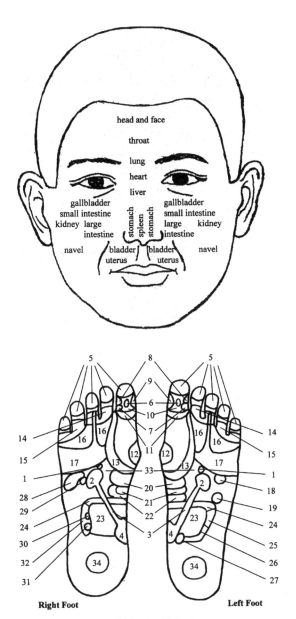

head and face

throat

lung

heart

liver

gallbladder   gallbladder
small intestine   small intestine
kidney   large   stomach   stomach   large   kidney
    intestine   spleen   intestine

navel   bladder   bladder   navel
     uterus   uterus

Right Foot   **Left Foot**

1. Adrenal gland
2. Kidney
3. Ureter
4. Bladder
5. Sinus
6. Pituitary gland
7. Brain stem
8. Trigeminal nerve
9. Nose
10. Head
11. Neck
12. Parathyroid glands
13. Thyroid gland
14. Eye
15. Ear
16. Trapezoid muscle
17. Lung and bronchus
18. Heart
19. Spleen
20. Stomach
21. Pancreas
22. Duodenum
23. Small intestine
24. Transverse colon
25. Descending colon
26. Rectum
27. Anus
28. Liver
29. Gallbladder
30. Appendix
31. Ileocaecal valve
32. Ascending colon
33. Solar plexus
34. Sex glands

Soles of Feet

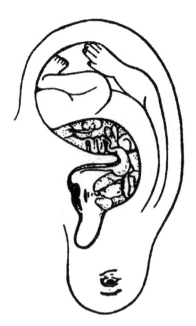

Ear Hologram of Body (above), Ear Acupoints (below)

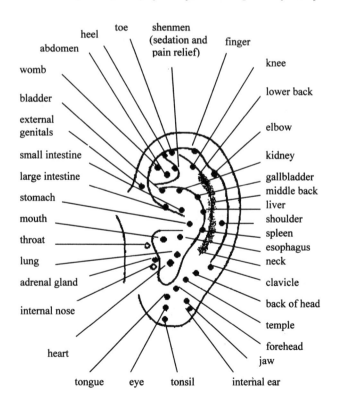

heel   toe   shenmen (sedation and pain relief)

abdomen   finger

womb

knee

bladder

lower back

external genitals

elbow

small intestine

kidney

large intestine

gallbladder

middle back

stomach

liver

mouth

shoulder

throat

spleen

esophagus

lung

neck

adrenal gland

clavicle

internal nose

back of head

temple

heart

forehead

jaw

tongue   eye   tonsil   internal ear

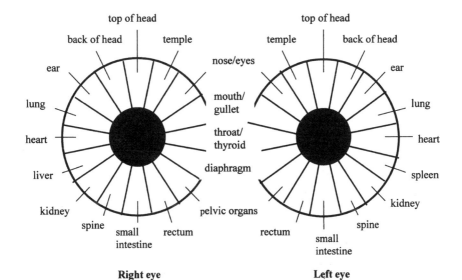

Iris of Eyes as Holograms of Body

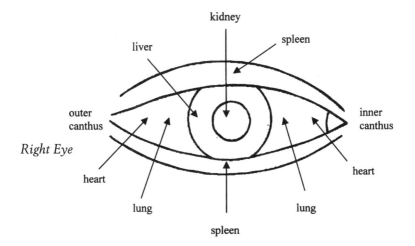

Right Eye

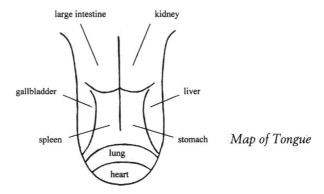

Map of Tongue

water and fire, dampness and dryness, heat and cold, and circulation and stagnation in the different organs. How does this internal climate of continual change balance out? Nature has found a way that allows for endless fluctuations of energy and yet gives stability to the living system. When we get overheated, for instance, we need water to cool us down. After heavy physical work, we need to take a rest. When we get too emotional, we need to find peace.

These simple examples show that we live with rhythms that shape our lives. They are found everywhere in nature, too; night follows day, the tides flow with the phases of the moon, the seasons come and go. All life on earth depends on such rhythms. If we listen to our bodily rhythms, we will soon detect the ebb and flow of many subtle changes that are going on all the time within us. We won't notice unless we pay special attention because the pace of life today is not geared to these biorhythms.

Have you ever had the experience of lying in bed at night with your mind racing, unable to switch it off, and then finding that when you do sleep, you wake during the night with disturbing dreams, or in a sweat? Enjoying deep and restful sleep is essential to good health. We know from medical research that if we don't get enough sleep, the stress on the body leads to lasting hormonal and chemical changes that can cause disease.

The natural rhythm of the body is to rest at least twice during the twenty-four hour cycle, not just at night but also in the middle of the day. Consider some of the ancient civilizations of the world— China, India, and Greece—which all developed a tradition of midday rest. By contrast in modern industrialized societies, we tend to work nonstop till evening; then we rest. In fact, most of us are overtired, though not always conscious of it. To keep going, we take caffeine or alcohol and watch stimulating programs on television while "relaxing." By the time we go to bed, our bodies are profoundly out of balance.

To understand the fundamental principle of nature's energy balance, we will next examine the *taiji*, the Chinese symbol of *yin* and *yang*, to see how body rhythms work day and night.

Yin and *Yang*:
Nature's Energy Balance

The Dao begot one.
One begot two.
Two begot three.
And three begot the ten thousand things.

The ten thousand things carry yin and embrace yang.
They achieve harmony by combining these forces.

—Laozi, *Daodejing*

CONSIDER the ancient Chinese *taiji* symbol (see page 12), which describes the fundamental dynamic balance of the whole universe. As noted earlier, the universe is organized like one giant hologram. The *taiji* reminds us that this holds true at every level of magnification, from the cosmos right down to the micro-universe of the human body.

The shaded area of the symbol represents *yin* and the white area *yang*. These two energies are opposing in nature but have a complementary relationship and are always found together. There are endless examples: sun and moon, earth and sky, fire and water, light and shade, hard and soft. Human properties are also attributed to these energies; *yang* as the active, male principle and *yin* as the receptive, female principle.

The *taiji* symbol describes both structure and function. It represents not only the building blocks of how everything is con-

11

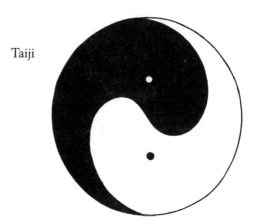

Taiji

structed but also how one half acts on the other to give rise to the movement and rhythm of life.

To look at structure first, consider the illustration of the *taiji* hierarchy. Note that *yang* is always present in *yin* and vice versa. Take the case of the human embryo. At the start, its physical anatomy is the same for both sexes. Then, in accordance with its genetic inheritance, the hormones it produces cause it to develop into

Taiji
*Hierarchy of
Forms*

Cosmos

Human beings

Internal organs

Individual cells

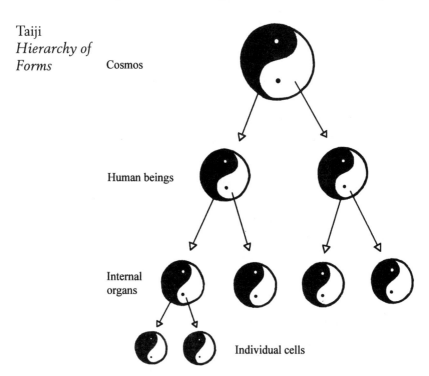

a boy *(yang)* or girl *(yin)*. *Yin* and *yang* are also expressed in the capacity of the male for receptivity *(yin)* and the capacity of the female for activity *(yang)*. All the internal organs of the body, as well
as the meridians, have a specific balance of *yin* and *yang* in order to
maintain health. Later we will discuss how health problems arise
when the balance is not maintained.

Turning now to function, we can understand the *taiji* symbol as
a "snapshot" of the movement of *qi* as it flows throughout the twenty-
four hour cycle of night and day. To understand how *yin* and *yang*
flow together, imagine you are standing on the edge of the circle at
11:00 A.M. Note that while most of the energy is *yang* like a bright
and sunny day, *yin* is just starting to grow. So it is not right just to
think of *yang* as day and *yin* as night, because it is in the middle of the
day that *yin* is born. In ancient Daoist texts, including the *Yijing*, the
moment of the arising of *yin* is called *shaoyin* (little *yin*). Here we
refer to this as the birth of baby *yin* to highlight the life-giving nature
of the cycle.

In China it is considered very important to have a period of rest

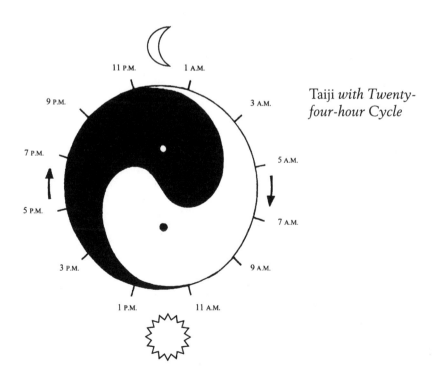

Taiji *with Twenty-
four-hour* Cycle

during baby *yin* time, between eleven and one o'clock. After eating, people lie down and have a nap. This ensures that baby *yin* is nourished from the start and helped to grow, for by giving it a good start, like a well-cared-for baby, it will grow steadily bigger and stronger over the coming twelve hours.

Now go around the circle to 11:00 P.M. In China, people consider it essential to be in bed by this hour, resting or sleeping. You can see that *yin* has become dominant, which means that body and mind are intended to be at peace, in accordance with the rhythm of the universe.

Next, see how between 11:00 P.M. and 1:00 A.M., although *yin* is still dominant, baby *yang* is born and then steadily grows through the first half of the day. During sleep, we not only benefit from the flow of *yin*, but also nourish baby *yang*, so that *yang qi* will grow strong and vigorous for the demands of the busy day ahead.

Take one more look at the *taiji*. As *yin* and *yang* embrace each other, right in the heart of *yin* there is an "eye" of *yang*, and likewise, in the *yang* an "eye" of *yin*. These eyes represent the seeds of energy that drive the cycle of *yin* and *yang* in its circular movement and highlight the fundamental principle that in *yang* there is always to be found *yin*, and within *yin, yang*.

There are two ways of picturing the circular motion of the *taiji*. Earlier we used the image of walking clockwise around the edge of the circle. Now picture standing still and imagine the *taiji* rotating around its center point, turning counterclockwise in a complete circle once every twenty-four hours. The effect reminds us that we are not looking at a stationary object but at a moving current of energy that flows without ceasing.

In the cosmos, there is no up and down, top and bottom. There is only a flow of energy. Here the *taiji* is shown with *yin* above and *yang* below for a reason that will be evident later when we discuss how *yin* and *yang qi* flow through the body. Next let us look in more detail at the meridians, the energy channels that were briefly mentioned.

The Meridians

All things arise from the Dao.
They are nourished by Virtue.
They are formed from matter.
They are shaped by environment.
Thus the ten thousand things all respect Dao and honor Virtue.
Respect of Dao and honor of Virtue are not demanded,
But they are in the nature of things.

—Laozi, *Daodejing*

THE MERIDIANS are a network of energy channels running throughout the entire body. We may picture them as a kind of road map, with twelve major meridians serving as the motorways, eight additional meridians like major trunk roads, and twelve divergent meridians like minor roads running alongside the motorways. Flowing out from all these meridians like a network of country lanes are small branches called collaterals.

The meridians do not figure in the anatomy of the body according to conventional western science, since they are not solid structures like arteries, veins, lymph ducts, or even nerves. Yet more than two thousand years ago, certain practitioners of Chinese medicine developed the art of "x-ray vision" through the skill of working directly with *qi* and described these "rivers of energy" in detail.

The ability to work with *qi* is called *qigong* in Chinese (the word "*gong*" meaning skill) and comes from an esoteric tradition that lies at the heart of Daoist and Buddhist teachings. Through the cultivation of special meditation techniques, the practitioner overcomes the

15

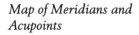

Map of Meridians and
Acupoints

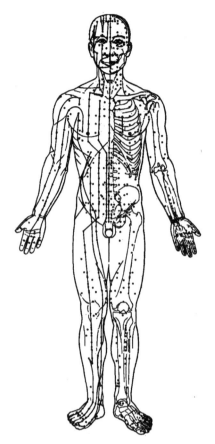

limits of ordinary sense perception and develops extraordinary powers. These include mastery over mind and matter to such a degree
that paranormal phenomena, as they are known in the West, are experienced and utilized in everyday life. This is how the leading doctors of Chinese medicine first observed the flow of subtle energies in
the body, for these practitioners were accomplished *qigong* masters.

Over the last twenty years, scientists have begun to investigate
the meridians using electrical conduction techniques. Research demonstrates that not only do meridians exist, they correspond exactly to
what *qigong* masters have been "seeing" for more than two millennia.

The flow of *qi* within the meridians is deeply connected to fluctuations in the energy of the sun, moon, earth, and stars. When we
see how powerful the effect of the moon is in producing the tides, it
is not surprising that the body itself can be affected, because the body

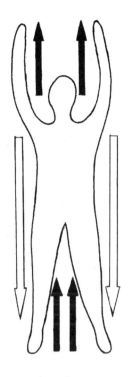

The Six Rising *Yin* Meridians:

lung
pericardium
heart
liver
spleen
kidney

Six Yin *and Six* Yang *Meridians*

The Six Descending *Yang* Meridians:

large intestine
triple burner
small intestine
stomach
gallbladder
bladder

is eighty-five percent water. The gravitational pull of the moon causes the *qi* in the meridians to rise, and where there is already emotional imbalance, the rise will be even greater as increasing *qi* stimulates the system.

A more gradual change is brought about by the four seasons. In summer, *qi* rises up to the surface of the skin. In winter, it runs deeper. Every acupuncturist knows that this change will affect the depth to which needles must be inserted into the body to find the meridians.

When we stand with our arms stretching upward, we stand between earth and heaven. According to the Daoist tradition, this is our place in the cosmos. In this posture, in the small cosmos of the body, *qi* flows in accordance with universal law. All six *yin* meridians of the body flow upward and all the six *yang* meridians flow downward, just as moist air *(yin)* rises and warmth of the sun *(yang)* radiates down on us.

The *taiji* illustration identifies the twelve major meridians. Each meridian plays its part throughout the twenty-four-hour cycle in

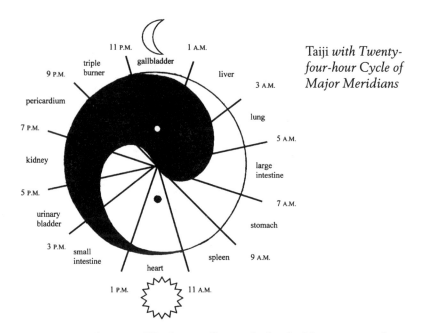

Taiji *with Twenty-four-hour Cycle of Major Meridians*

maintaining the overall balance of *qi* in the body. However, each meridian in turn passes through a phase of maximum sensitivity lasting about two hours, during which the flow of *qi* is concentrated in that meridian.

We shall now look at two of these meridians in more detail and discuss their function in both health and illness.

The Heart Meridian

You can see from the illustration that this meridian has three main branches running from the heart. One branch goes down to the small intestine, one branch to the throat, mouth, eye, and brain, and one branch to the lung, then down the inside of the arm to the tip of the little finger.

The heart itself functions overall as a *yang* organ. TCM visualizes it as a "fire organ" associated with activity and heat. During heart meridian time, between 11:00 A.M. and 1:00 P.M., it is tempting to exploit this readily available *yang* energy. Many people do just that by taking working lunches day after day. Yet heart meridian time deserves special attention because it is intimately linked

Heart Meridian

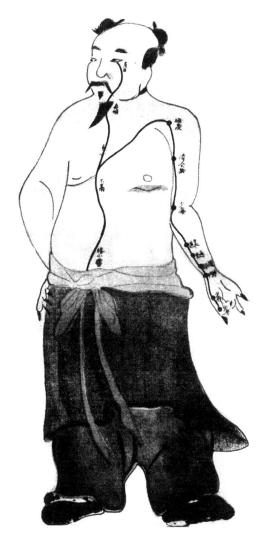

with the birth of baby *yin*, which the Chinese picture as drops of cool liquid. Although all meridians are concerned with the flow of both *yin* and *yang*, the heart meridian is defined as a *yin* meridian because of its role in the birth of baby *yin*.

When baby *yin* has been nourished by taking a rest during heart meridian time, the *qi* flows strongly in the heart meridian, with the result that the digestive system works well, the mind is alert and the eyes are bright, concentration and memory are enhanced, and the rhythm of sleep is deep and regular. The lungs will be healthy

Nourishing Baby Yin *and*
Baby Yang

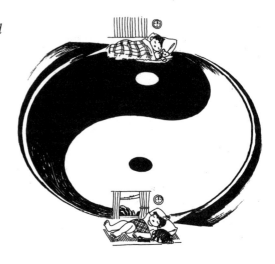

and the arms strong. In TCM, the lungs in turn control the skin, so that the condition of the skin, too, will be good.

In contrast, if no rest period is taken, the long-term consequences of *yin* deficiency can be serious. These include palpitations; pain around the heart; insomnia; excess sweating, especially at night; overheating of the palms and soles; arthritis; thirst; mouth ulcers; dryness of eyes; and intolerance of light. Other possible effects are itchy skin, headache, anxiety and depression, loss of concentration and memory, restlessness, and irritability.

In some countries, the lunch break is usually between 1:00 and 2:00 P.M., during small intestine meridian time. An earlier lunch hour is preferable, but if this cannot be managed, it is still better to rest between 1:00 and 2:00 P.M. than to go without.

After baby *yin* has been born, it is important to nurture *yin* carefully by refraining from too much vigorous activity and excitement in the second half of the day. **Whereas *yang* energy is given over to "doing," the character of *yin* is that of "being."** We shall see what this means in practice in Part Four of this book.

Since the meridians carry both *yin* and *yang*, it is not surprising that symptoms also arise when the heart meridian is deficient in *yang*. This happens either because baby *yang* has not been nourished at night or because the reserves of *yang* have been exhausted through excess activity. More often than not, it is caused by a mixture of both.

We will examine the birth of baby *yang* during the night when discussing the gallbladder meridian. As to the exhaustion of *yang qi* during the day, bear in mind that because the first half of the day is *yang* time, people often feel energetic and get carried away with the challenge of tasks needing to be done and the excitement of interacting with other people. If *yang qi* is weak to start with, working straight through lunchtime makes further demands on it. The result is that the heart meridian *yang* becomes inflamed and burns out. Because the body's warning system has been masked by overactivity, damage takes place without awareness of what is going wrong. The list of problems which can occur when *yang* is depleted is a long one: stiffness and pain around the neck and shoulders, bad breath, indigestion, irritable bowel syndrome, loss of voice, dizziness, weakness, fatigue, fainting, vomiting blood or losing blood in stools or urine, heavy and irregular menstruation, shortness of breath, discoloration of nails, overexcitement, impulsiveness, agitation, and irrationality.

We have dealt with the problems of *yin* and *yang* in the heart meridian separately here in order to describe how the two energy patterns coexist. In everyday life, however, when the *qi* in the meridian has been affected, both *yin* and *yang* are likely to be disturbed and so the picture is often a mixed one with a combination of symptoms.

The Gallbladder Meridian

The gallbladder meridian starts at the outer corner of the eye, goes to the ear, runs back and forth over the scalp and then down the length of the body to the hip, continues down the outside of the leg, and ends between the fourth and fifth toes. The gallbladder meridian is very important because it is linked to baby *yang*. If you refer to the picture of *taiji* with meridians (see page 18) you will understand its importance, since gallbladder meridian time is between 11:00 p.m. and 1:00 a.m., when baby *yang* is born.

When baby *yang* is well nourished, sleep is sound and undisturbed. The body is warm and comfortable and you wake refreshed at an early hour, often at sunrise. The day begins with energy and

Gallbladder Meridian

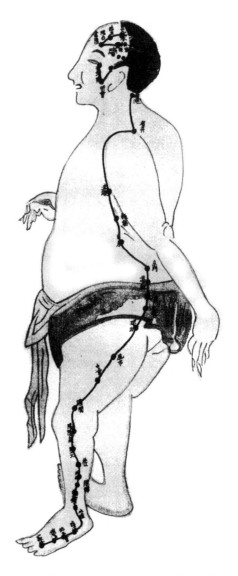

vitality because *yang qi* has been steadily growing stronger throughout the night. You get out of bed not because you must but because
your body is telling you it wants to get started. This sensation of
well-being lasts through the whole day, provided *yang qi* is conserved by taking the lunchtime rest.

The more consistently this routine is followed, the greater are
the benefits. The immune system is strengthened and resistance is
developed to infections and other debilitating conditions such as

chronic fatigue syndrome. Muscle strength and tolerance of cold are increased, high blood pressure is reduced, and migraines, tension headaches, shoulder, neck, and back pain and stiffness are prevented.

On the other hand, if baby *yang* is not properly nourished, the consequences can be serious. The following problems are liable to occur: eye strain and visual disturbances, migraines, tension headache, tinnitus (ringing in the ears), hearing loss, facial paralysis (Bell's palsy), poor thermoregulation (tendency to fluctuate between hot and cold), and strains and pains in the musculoskeletal system.

Note that as the meridian travels down the body, it reaches around the side to lie under the rib cage, where it connects with the gallbladder and liver. Further along, the meridian goes through the hip joint before continuing down the leg. This is why when baby *yang* is weak there is a tendency to indigestion and gallbladder disease. Hip pain may be misdiagnosed as a joint problem while pain going down the leg can be mistaken for sciatica caused by a prolapsed disc.

The gallbladder meridian is highly sensitive to emotional upset. Both the gallbladder and the liver may be directly affected and again, because of the pathway of this meridian, incapacitating neck, back, and hip pain can develop. Back pain causes more lost work time than any other disorder; thus it is important both to nourish baby *yang* during the night and to maintain a calm and peaceful mind during the day.

All these symptoms can be avoided by tuning in to the rhythm of nature and harnessing the energy of the body to promote health and balance. The symptoms that arise are giving us a message about what we are doing wrong and how, at the deeper level, the problem has arisen.

The Flow of Q*i* in Nature

The great Dao flows everywhere, both to the left and to the right.
The ten thousand things depend upon it; it holds nothing back.
It fulfills its purpose silently and makes no claim.

It nourishes the ten thousand things,
And yet is not their lord.
It has no aim; it is very small.

The ten thousand things return to it,
Yet it is not their lord.
It is very great.

It does not show greatness, and is therefore truly great.

　　　　　　　　　—Laozi, *Daodejing*

WE HAVE SAID earlier that there is a special reason for putting *yin* on top and *yang* underneath in the *taiji* that can be understood with reference to the world of nature. The mountain rises up out of the lush vegetation of the valley below. Down the slopes trickle mountain streams. The earth at the foot of the mountain is rich and moist, and the warmth of the golden sunshine filters down through the trees and green plants that grow in profusion on the floor of the valley.

Up on the mountaintop the air is clear and cold. Way below in the valley it is warm and humid. Unseen, yet endlessly flowing from valley to mountaintop, are currents of air, warmed by the sun down in the valley and now climbing the mountainside. As the warm,

24

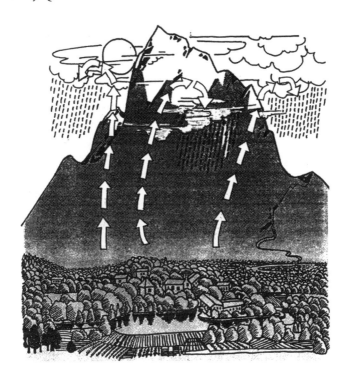

moist air ascends into the sky it begins to cool, and as it cools, drop-
lets of water vapor form. Mist and clouds condense out of the clear
air and wreathe the mountaintop. Light rain begins to fall on the
upper slopes, nourishing streams that carry the water back down to
the vegetation in the valley and the life there that it supports.

Now look again at the *taiji* illustration and visualize the sun
(yang) radiating down and warming the moist air in the valley *(yin)*
that is rising into the sky. Note how this interpretation of the *taiji*
compares with the picture of the human body showing the six *yang*

Taiji

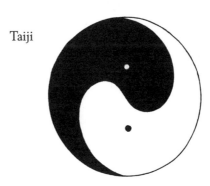

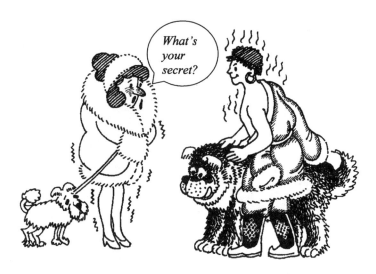

meridians descending and the six *yin* meridians rising (see page 17). The circulation of *qi* in the body follows the same pattern as in nature. There is one important difference: the human body is mobile and so its internal climate has to be protected. This is why people in China are careful to keep their feet warm by wearing socks and shoes and by bathing their feet in hot water before bed, while keeping the upper part of the body cool. Tibetans often leave the shoulder uncovered, even at high altitude, while at the same time wearing padded trousers and boots. This ensures good health, strength, and resistance to infections.

Yang without *yin* is a desert. *Yin* without *yang* is a dead sea. But *yin* and *yang* always act together, because their function is for each to be continually giving birth to the other. In the body, the *yang* aspect is the *qi*, and the *yin* is the blood. So the Chinese speak of "*qi* leading the blood," just as the warm rays of the sun activate life in the moisture of the valley. In the same breath, the Chinese refer to blood as the "mother of *qi*." *Yin* and *yang* are inseparable wherever life is to be found.

Harnessing Nature's Q*i:*
The Three *Dantian*

Force is followed by loss of strength
This is not the way of Dao.
That which goes against the Dao
Comes to an early end.

—Laozi, *Daodejing*

THE CONCEPT of the energy centers of the body can be traced to the ancient teachings of the Daoist school of Quanzhendao (Ultimate truth of the Dao). It was discovered that with regular *qigong* practice, energy flowed within the body in the vertical and horizontal planes. These planes intersected in three places—the head, chest, and abdomen—and where they crossed, intense foci of energy could be generated. These energy centers were called the three *dantian*—the lower *dantian* restoring *jing*, the energy essence of the reproductive organs; the middle *dantian* restoring *qi*, concerned with bodily and emotional energy; and the upper *dantian* restoring *shen*, or spirit. It is of note that in recent biophysics research, three energy centers have been identified that correspond to the location of the three *dantian*.

The Lower *Dantian*

You may have noticed that when you relax, your tummy gurgles, sometimes quite noisily. In the West, we regard this as embarrassing

27

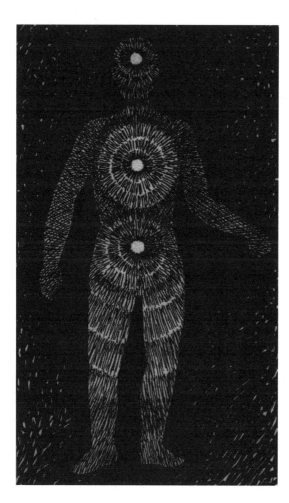

Three Dantian

and often apologize for it. In China, tummy gurgles are welcomed, for they simply mean that a natural bodily process is underway. Gurgles result from the movement of *qi*, which is activating the digestive process and converting food into pure energy, a transformation fundamental to life. A strong lower *dantian* ensures that the digestion releases yet more *qi*, which can be concentrated and stored in the abdomen. From here, the *qi* is used to power all the physical processes of the body. It is like the roots of a great tree that penetrate deep into the ground and draw up the nutrients from the soil. The roots also give stability, so that the tree can withstand gale force winds. In both *qigong* and yoga practice, special attention is given to abdominal breathing because it activates and strengthens this energy center.

The Middle *Dantian*

The middle *dantian* is situated within the chest cavity. It is linked with the heart and its emotions. One way to imagine it is to picture the trunk of a great tree. If the roots are deep, the trunk of the tree grows strong. The rising sap gives it the flexibility to sway with the wind and keeps the tree healthy throughout all the seasons of the year, regardless of rain, snow, or gales.

The drama of human existence requires us to cope with all kinds of emotional turbulence. If we are well rooted in our lower *dantian* and also have a strong middle *dantian*, our energy can spread throughout our whole being like the sap of the tree flowing to the tip of every branch. Then we can cope with the storms of life as well as enjoy the warmth of the sun and the beauty of our surroundings.

The Upper *Dantian*

Here we must leave the image of the tree, because the upper *dantian* relates to the function of consciousness, directing our thoughts and actions. It is located behind the eyes and is linked to the pineal gland, an outgrowth of the base of the brain now known to be concerned with the balance of many hormones. According to ancient texts, this region of the brain is responsible for the opening of the third eye. The Daoist and Buddhist traditions teach that this happens when we learn to live without greed, attachment, and desire. With regular *qigong* practice or meditation, we gain access to a higher level of consciousness or divine spirit, known as *shen*. *Shen* enables us to harmonize with the whole cosmos, our minds and bodies merging as one. With this expansion of consciousness, the tasks of daily life become effortless. Phenomena usually regarded as paranormal such as telepathy, precognition, clairvoyance, and perception of the human aura can be accessed at will. Most importantly for our daily health, when *shen* is strong, extraordinary healing of the body can take place. We are being guided from within by a deep wisdom that goes beyond time and space.

In health, the three *dantian* are balanced, and since *qi* flows freely between them they work as one. But if the lower *dantian* should be weak, no matter how great the vision and how powerful the will, the body will let us down, just as the tree with weak roots will die early. Physical disorders include deterioration of the immune system and cancer of the abdominal organs.

If the middle *dantian* is weak, the emotions of life overwhelm us, like a tree with a damaged trunk that cannot bear the weight of the branches when the wind blows. Heart attack from stress, or pneumonia following bereavement are just two such examples.

When the upper *dantian* is weak, the situation is like a car on the move with a driver who does not know how to use the controls. No matter how wonderful the car, it will be a menace to others, and before long the driver will damage both the car and himself! Disorders include emotional instability and the negative influences the mind can have on the body. Fear, anger, overexcitement, and stress all lead to psychosomatic problems or physical diseases such as high blood pressure and coronary artery disease.

The body has a mind of its own and the art is learning how to listen to what it is saying. Every symptom is a communication, alerting us to an underlying imbalance. This information is of immense benefit, for many disorders can be corrected with the help of nature's own medicine, already there within the body and simply waiting to be used.

PART TWO

The Information System of the Body

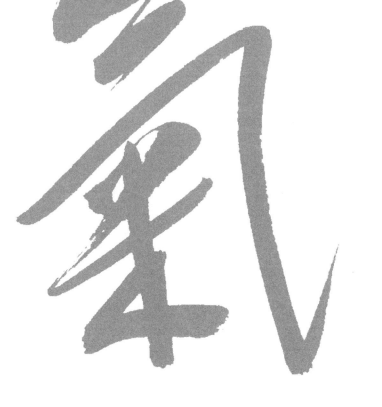

The Natural
Human Life Span

A man is born gentle and weak.
At his death he is hard and stiff.
Green plants are tender and filled with sap.
At their death they are withered and dry.

Therefore the stiff and unbending is the disciple of death.
The gentle and yielding is the disciple of life.

—Laozi, *Daodejing*

HERE FOLLOWS a remarkable story. It tells us what we can achieve, if only we live by the medicine that comes free with life itself and learn how to maintain the balance and harmony within us.

In the south part of China there is a remote village that was recently visited by a journalist. He arrived in the village while a wedding ceremony was taking place. Noisy festivities were going on and he inquired who was getting married. He was somewhat surprised to hear that the bride was eighty-two and the bridegroom was in his nineties. He was even more astonished to be told that marriages at this age were not unusual.

The average life span in this village is more than one hundred years. What is the secret of this longevity? The villagers lead a simple life, one that has changed little for thousands of years. They live very close to nature. There is no electricity, so villagers get up at sunrise and go to bed at sunset. They work together in the fresh air farming their crops and eating the fresh food from their own fields. Once a month they apply a traditional herb known in China as *aiye (Artemesia argyi)* to a special point on the stomach meridian by the process of moxibustion. Most important of all, the villagers live happy and peaceful lives. Everyone is contented with what they have and no one is greedy for more. Life is lived in accordance with nature's rhythms. It is a way of life established long ago, far removed from the hustle and bustle of what we take for normal in modern daily living.

We usually think of life in ancient times as primitive and dangerous, yet in China such communities had a wisdom that is lost to us today. There were no luxuries or labor-saving devices, but these people knew the importance of harmony of body and mind, and with the right balance of exercise and rest maintained a consistently high level of *qi*. As a result, their bodies were strong and resistant to infection and they could take in their stride adverse living conditions, such as cold and damp, that would have us reaching for the electric blanket.

When we take care of the body, we discover that it is a powerful force indeed, with capacities far beyond our usual expectations. Another illustration of the body's power concerns the Buddhist monk Haiyu. He was born in Beijing in 1513 and spent a life of absolute simplicity in a cave on Jiuhua Mountain, where he lived on herbs and mountain fruit, eating only twice a week, and spent his time writing Buddhist manuscripts and practicing *qigong*.

In 1623, at the age of 110, Haiyu decided it was time to die. He left letters giving the exact day and time of his death. Three years later, his body was found perfectly preserved, as if he were still meditating in the lotus position. His body was moved to the temple, where it can still be viewed today.

Longevity is the subject of speculation in the West, and lively centenarians are sometimes interviewed on radio or television. Some put their good health down to a daily tot of spirits and others to home remedies like cloves and garlic. What is striking about all these people is their happiness and contentment, which has given them a wonderful sense of moderation in all things and a relish for the simple pleasures of life.

We need to confront what it is that most of us are doing to our-selves to cut short our lives so drastically. Many people look de-pressed and worn out by the time they reach fifty, when this need be no more than half the journey and with some of the best years still ahead. We can be thankful for the many advances in western medi-cine that have occurred in the last fifty years. The average life span has increased for males from sixty-six to seventy-four and for fe-males from seventy to eighty. But when it comes to the science of aging, we need to look further afield, for this increase in the average life span is largely due to the fact that death from disease in the younger age groups, especially infancy and childhood, has been greatly reduced. What the statistics also show is that in the older age groups, cancer and diseases of the lungs and circulatory system have actually increased. **Once the age of sixty-five years has been suc-cessfully attained, the average remaining life span has remained unchanged in fifty years of medical science.**

How can we improve on this? The answer is found in five thousand years of wisdom that teaches us that our bodies already know what we need to do to reach our full potential. Provided we learn how to tune in to these needs and respond appropriately, with calmness and a daily routine that respects the natural flow of *yin* and *yang*, our health is safeguarded by the *qi* of the cosmos even if we are surrounded by the hurly-burly of city life.

Recognizing the Signals
Your Body Sends

Man follows the earth.
Earth follows heaven.
Heaven follows the Dao.
Dao follows what is natural.

—Laozi, *Daodejing*

MODERN SCIENCE has shown the physical body to be a miracle of living engineering. But there is another miracle, less tangible but no less real, that has been known about in China for thousands of years. **The body is not just made up of visible matter that can be viewed under the microscope or analyzed in test tubes. Its fundamental structure is made of *qi*, just as everything in the physical universe is made of *qi*.**

At the deepest level, *qi* is a unity that cannot be described in words. It is the source of all creation. At the next level, in the familiar world of our five senses, *qi* exists in everything we touch, smell, taste, see, and hear.

In the East, people are content to accept that *qi* is a unity, and they don't try to analyze it into various components. But since the aim of this book is to draw out and highlight those manifestations of *qi* essential to our understanding of health and illness, it is useful to consider how *qi* functions in several ways:

• **As energy, *qi* is like an underground river.** It flows without ceasing throughout the whole body and in health it moves si-

36

lently, harmonizing and balancing body processes second by second.

- **As information, *qi* works like radio signals endlessly being transmitted and received.** It is like a program going out on the BBC that takes live feedback from the listeners. In this case BBC stands for "body broadcasting center." Whenever a problem arises in the body, there is an immediate broadcast that reveals the underlying disturbance provided the message is received and understood.

- **The *qi* that surrounds us all can conveniently be called environment-*qi*.** We have discussed how the body works like a hologram so that each body part contains a map of the whole body. But remember that at a higher level of magnification, the body houses a map of the whole universe! This is why *qi* travels between people, as well as throughout the whole of nature, and we shall look later at how one person's *qi* can affect another, for good or ill.

A healthy body feels calm, relaxed, and strong. Body movements are light and accurate, made without strain or effort. The body is looking after itself so well the owner doesn't need to be aware of it doing its job. This is because the energy-*qi* is full and well balanced throughout the whole body. Put another way, the underground river flows swift, strong, and silent. At such times there is no need for news broadcasts because there is no bad news to tell and no corrective action required. When you listen in, what you experience is the background music of energy, lightness, and happiness welling up from within the self. It only remains to dive into the river of *qi* and float peacefully with the current.

A word of warning! In this relaxed state, it might seem to others that you are daydreaming. You may feel in a bit of a trance and it is true that it takes time to learn how to adjust to this in your daily life. When you do adjust, you find that you are in fact highly efficient. Your intelligence is more focused, your concentration is heightened, your memory is enhanced, and your creativity surges.

Uroboros

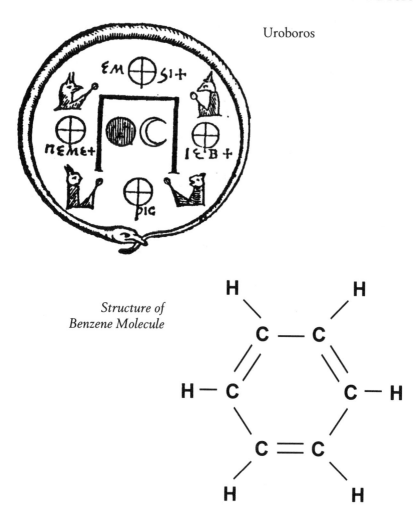

Structure of Benzene Molecule

Many of the greatest discoveries of science owe their invention to this dreamy state of mind. Thomas Edison, who invented the light bulb, found that his most brilliant ideas came to him when he sat still in a state of deep relaxation. He would take a handful of metal ball bearings and hold them over a dish. When he relaxed to the point of sleep, the ball bearings would fall into the dish, rousing him to pick them up again. Friedrich Kekule, the famous chemist, struggled for months to understand the structure of the benzene molecule. Deep in reverie, the image came to him of a snake with its tail in its mouth (the ancient symbol known as the *uroboros*). This vision instantly solved the problem for him; he saw that carbon atoms form rings, and this breakthrough formed the basis of all modern organic chemistry.

All of us can benefit from the creative potential of relaxation. Contemporary research has shown that deep relaxation enhances concentration and learning. In China, seventy-one college students were taught to practice *qigong* for twenty minutes daily for three months. Their scores on mathematics improved by 14 percent and on languages by 50 percent. Experienced *qigong* practitioners are known to have exceptional powers of the mind, with heightened vision and hearing extending to extrasensory perception, and total control of body physiology such as pulse and blood pressure. In the state of deep relaxation the whole wisdom of the universe flows in like a waterfall, and learning and creativity become effortless. This state is called *ding neng sheng hui* (wisdom within calmness).

In contrast, when the body is not in balance and we are tired and drained, the river of *qi* does not flow as it should. It may be depleted, in which case the current will be sluggish. Our limbs feel weary, we start yawning, and there is dryness of the eyes, all of which result from the lack of nourishment of *qi*.

These bodily reactions are among the first of the news broadcasts to go on air. If we take a break then and there and wait till the river of energy-*qi* rises, we quickly find ourselves refreshed and the symptoms will disappear. Unfortunately, all too often we respond by pouring ourselves another cup of coffee, overriding the signals our information-*qi* is sending and paying the price later. When we ignore these early warning signals, the body tries to warn us by sending stronger messages such as increasing fatigue, tension, loss of concentration, headache, irritability, itching, flushing hot and cold, aches and pains, and an unusual degree of clumsiness.

As the level of *qi* continues to fall, the body tries to compensate for the deficiency by using muscle pumps to drive the *qi* along. This is why tension arises in the muscles. Temporarily there may be an improvement, but in time the level falls so low that only a sluggish flow of *qi* remains. Circulation of *qi* to the upper part of the body will be particularly affected, hence the loss of concentration. Because the passage of *qi* through the skin is now so slow, itching is a common symptom.

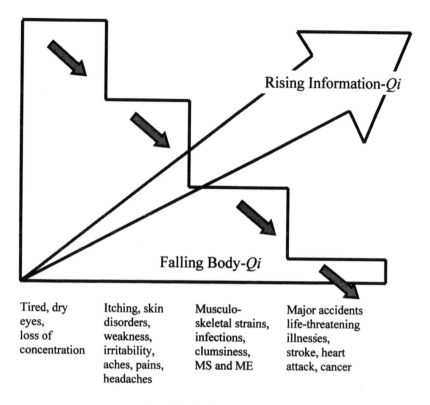

Rising Information-*Qi*

Falling Body-*Qi*

| Tired, dry eyes, loss of concentration | Itching, skin disorders, weakness, irritability, aches, pains, headaches | Musculo-skeletal strains, infections, clumsiness, MS and ME | Major accidents life-threatening illnesses, stroke, heart attack, cancer |

*Graph of Information-*Qi

When the *qi* stagnates, toxic wastes build up and cause aching. If the current of *qi* finds itself completely blocked at a particular location, it tries to force a way through in an effort to keep flowing. This produces a throbbing sensation or sharp pain if the *qi* is still strong, or a dull ache if the *qi* is weak.

If we still don't respond to the warnings coming through, we are at risk of serious problems. For example, when we suppress a headache with a painkiller and then carry on as if it hadn't happened, we are covering up damage that has already begun. We become vulnerable to heavy colds, joint pains, muscle and ligament strains, and skin disorders. As time goes on, the immune system deteriorates, resulting in chronic infections and inflammatory disorders such as chronic fatigue syndrome and multiple sclerosis.

NATURE OF SYMPTOM	STATE OF *QI*	STATE OF BLOOD	ENERGETIC PROCESS
FIXED SHARP PAIN	STILL STRONG AND MOVING	SEVERE STAGNATION	STRONG *QI* TRYING TO FORCE ITS WAY THROUGH BLOCK
FIXED DULL ACHE	WEAK	STAGNATION	WEAK *QI* CANNOT FORCE THROUGH BLOCK
MOVING SHARP PAIN	STRONG BUT INTERMITTENT	STAGNATION	*QI* FORCES WITH DIFFICULTY THROUGH A NUMBER OF BLOCKS
MOVING DULL ACHE	WEAK	INTERMITTENT STAGNATION	WEAK *QI* FORCES ITS WAY THROUGH ISLANDS OF RESISTANCE

Signs of Blocked Qi

At the most serious level of disturbance, we have ignored the warning signals to such an extent that we can no longer hear them at all. We have lost the ability to tune in to the underlying problem. All the body can do to force us to pay attention is to shout disaster from the rooftops. We fall victim to major accidents or develop life-threatening diseases such as cancer or heart disease.

The body is now in a state of life-threatening crisis. But such a crisis can be a turning point in life. The Chinese word for crisis is "*weiji.*" "*Wei*" means disaster, but "*ji*" means opportunity. The changes that need to be made will be deep and far-reaching. Here the message is simple yet profound: "Give up your old way of life and start a new one!"

Case Studies from a
Specialist Clinic

Knowing ignorance is strength.
Ignoring knowledge is sickness.

—Laozi, *Daodejing*

THIJ **CHAPTER** describes a number of cases of serious illness or disability that help link theory to practice and illustrate how the concepts discussed so far are applied in specialist treatment.

The Body's Warning Signals Ignored

A fifty-year-old woman complained of a red, itchy rash on her abdomen and chest. The rash had been present for a few weeks. She was also tender over the neck, shoulders, and the middle of the chest, which in TCM are typical signs of emotional stress. She added that she had recently fallen over, twice within three days, and was suffering from headaches and back, knee, and ankle pains. Questioned, she admitted that her bowel movements were giving her trouble, with bouts of constipation and diarrhea.

On TCM examination, her "sea of *qi*" level was extremely low. This is an acupoint in the lower *dantian* situated below the navel. When the *qi* is strong, pressing on this point meets with a springy resistance, but when it is weak, the fingers easily go in, as if encountering an empty space, and in extreme cases the spine can easily be touched.

Soon the whole picture emerged. This woman had been under strain for several months due to pressures at home. Initially she had felt tired, but with so much to do she did not ease up. Next she caught a cold, which she tried to ignore. Her sleep became disturbed by night sweats; she began to get headaches, and within a few weeks developed symptoms of an irritable bowel. At the same time, her skin began itching and red patches appeared. The climax to her misfortune came with her falls. On each occasion she tripped and landed heavily on her back. Now she had strains and bruises to contend with in addition to her other problems.

She was treated with acupressure, acupuncture, and *qigong*, and immediately fell into a profound sleep. She was wakened after three quarters of an hour and found herself free of pain. The rash disappeared after three treatments, her bowel movements returned to normal, and she reported feeling her old self again.

This case, which is typical of many, highlights the inner language of the body. The various symptoms this patient suffered were due to the signals of information-*qi* getting louder as time went on, warning her to slow down as her energy-*qi* continued to decline. The crisis culminated in her accidents due to clumsiness, and she was finally forced to take a break.

The immediate effect of treatment had been to restore the patient's *qi*. But equally important was the advice given by the doctor, who pointed out what had been happening to her body so that she would know how to take better care of herself next time.

Live Now, Pay Later

Here is an example of just how serious the long-term consequences can be when *qi* is not maintained during the whole of a person's adult life.

A forty-year-old woman came to the clinic to see if TCM could help her thyroid disorder. She had experienced symptoms of an overactive thyroid gland for about one year. The medical diagnosis had been confirmed after six months and since then medication had partially suppressed thyroid function, though not sufficiently. The patient continued to experience palpitations, sweats, poor sleep, restlessness, and headaches, as well as exophthalmia (abnormally protruding eyes).

On TCM examination, striking findings included an empty "sea of *qi*," indicating serious weakness of the lower *dantian*. The tongue was large and pale, revealing *qi* and blood deficiency, with a yellow, sticky coating caused by "damp heat." (This symptom occurs when the *qi* can no longer maintain a fresh circulation of body fluids, which then begin overheating.) The pulse was fast and shallow, suggesting "fire rising." (This means that *qi* is not stabilized within the *dantian* but is escaping onto the surface of the body.) Both feet were icy cold to the touch.

The circulation of the hands and feet are especially important in TCM because the major meridians start and end in the fingertips or toes. In "The Flow of Q*i* in Nature," we explained how healthy living depends on keeping the feet warm and the head cool. We used the example of how warmth at the foot of the mountain brought the valley to life. So nature intended it to be with the human body. Yet think of how often in western culture people walk around in all weathers with cold hands, bare legs, and with nothing but thin shoes on their feet. In contrast, the top half of the body is usually warmly covered. According to TCM, this is why arthritis is so common, as well as headaches and full-blown migraines, for the cold directly affects the meridians and freezes the flow of *qi*.

This patient's case illustrates what we call the the volcano effect. The body takes emergency action to get the *qi* flowing, but because the flow of *qi* to the lower half of the body is blocked, the pressure builds up in the top half like a volcano. In this case, the consequence was headaches, protruding eyes, sweats, and palpitations, while the lower limbs and feet remained cold.

Asked about her lifestyle, the patient revealed some highly relevant information. This was a woman who did not know how to rest and who had been in overdrive all her working life. Even when her second child was born eight years previously, she had gone back to work within forty-eight hours to carry on managing her business. Her expectation was that she must always feel as energetic as when she was twenty, and so she went on making enormous demands of herself.

Overactivity is, of course, typical of thyrotoxicosis (overactive thyroid). From the TCM perspective, this woman had put herself under such pressure for so many years that her body had no choice but to try to live up to the demands she was making on it. Her thyroid gland began to overact in order to compensate for her deficient *qi*. If she had understood the serious nature of the signals her body was sending her, she could have set about changing her lifestyle. This never occurred to her. After having her babies, for instance, her only thought was that she must get back to work.

In China, it is traditional for the new mother to rest for at least fifty-six days following childbirth. Only family members are allowed to visit and the mother does not go out of the house for the first month. Because body-*qi* has been depleted and needs building up, she must protect herself from any environment-*qi* which could harm her, such as cold, damp, wind, or excess heat. Baths and showers are avoided because the body cannot cope with sudden temperature changes. Food and drink must be warmed, and when the mother first goes outside, she is wrapped from tip to toe in warm clothing, making her easily recognizable in the street as a new mother.

In the case under discussion, the patient received acupuncture and herbs over a period of eighteen months. Her sleep improved and the palpitations stopped. She noted that the sensation of pressure behind her eyes improved when she rested and her swollen thyroid gland became visibly smaller.

The Ring That Changed a Woman's Life

A fifty-year-old woman came to the clinic suffering from dizziness and fainting spells over a fifteen-year period. She had been extensively examined, including studies of heart function and brain waves, but all findings were normal. Typically, she would feel dizzy on waking in the morning, and when getting out of bed or stretching, turning,

Small Intestine Meridian

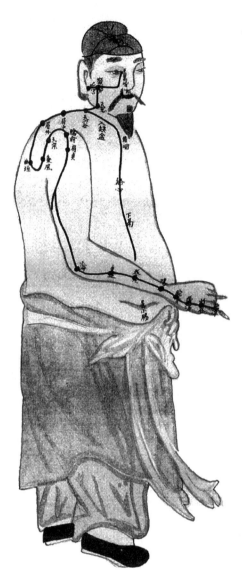

or bending over, she was liable to faint without warning. At first the fainting spells were every two or three months, but the condition had steadily progressed so that she had been forced to give up golf, her favorite recreation. Fainting was now occurring daily, and she dared not go out in public.

Before TCM examination, the patient was asked to take off the ring from her little finger, for it was obviously too tight. The patient replied that she couldn't possibly do that, because she had put this ring on at age nineteen and had never taken it off since. Now it was stuck fast!

On TCM examination, the internal organs all appeared normal. This did not surprise the doctor, who then told the patient that the ring had to be cut off. The patient was somewhat surprised but did as she was told. When she came back to the clinic the next week, she was all smiles. There had been no dizziness or fainting and she had already been out on the golf course, for the first time in fifteen years.

What was the secret of this success? It was all due to restoring the flow of *qi* to the heart meridian. This meridian, which extends down the inner side of the little finger to the tip (see page 19), had become blocked over the years by the pressure of the ring.

The small intestine meridian goes down the outside of the little finger and if similarly obstructed can give rise to symptoms of pain in the shoulder and neck, tinnitus, and stomach upset. Since meridians run along every finger, it is best to wear no rings. If rings are worn, it is essential that they be comfortable and easily removable. They should always be taken off at night.

The Engineer Who Ran out of Steam

Chronic fatigue syndrome, also known as myalgic encephalitis or ME, is the subject of much current medical research in the West. It is a condition that responds very well, and often rapidly, to TCM.

A forty-five-year-old engineer complained of feeling unwell, with headaches, dizziness, tinnitus, and a continuing sensation of extreme tiredness. His limbs were weak and aching and he explained that if he rested for a day (which he was reluctant to do, being self-employed) he felt better, though the following day he would feel just as tired as ever. He also mentioned that his bowels were upset, alternately loose and constipated.

Closer study of his background revealed that he had first felt unwell about one year before with a heavy cold, at a time when he was under pressure at work. Since he thought that a mere cold should not stop him from working, he carried on as usual. The symptoms of dizziness and tiredness started soon after. He consulted his family doctor who prescribed medication, which helped for a short while. Then the symptoms worsened again and although he struggled to keep going at work over the next year, he finally had to admit defeat.

On TCM examination, his tongue was found to be enlarged and pale with indentations (teethmarks) around the edge of the tongue, a sign of long-term spleen *qi* deficiency. The lower *dantian* was empty and the kidney meridian was very weak. Needles were inserted into the "sea of *qi*" and along the kidney meridians on both sides. The patient fell asleep at once.

After the treatment, the problem of *qi* deficiency was explained to him as being like a water storage tank that had emptied, a comparison he readily understood. Catching the severe cold in the first place was a sign that the water level had already fallen very low. Although since then water had been trickling in, in his condition it was like trying to run a bath before the tank had been given enough time to fill, for each time it would immediately run dry again. This is why, although he felt better after a day of rest, the exhaustion would return, as it so often does in this disorder, as soon as he got going again the following day.

When asked about the dizziness and tinnitus, the doctor explained that the body is like a building. If the water pressure falls, the water cannot be pumped up to the upper story. The lower *dantian* works both as a reservoir for *qi* and as a pumping station that sends the *qi* up to the head. Dizziness and tinnitus are liable to occur when *qi* levels are low.

The patient stayed off work for the next week and came for a second treatment. He reported that the dizziness and tinnitus had greatly improved and that he had already noticed much more energy. Because he was already feeling so much better, he was keen to get back to work. Within a week he had relapsed and further treatment was needed.

He now wanted to know if he would ever completely recover. The answer was yes, but with a proviso. He was going to have to learn how to maintain his *qi*. The doctor reminded him that he had fallen ill in the first place because, without realizing it, he had been running on low *qi*. Since that time, his *qi* had never had the chance to return to normal. How quickly the level would rise would depend on the patient. If he took the necessary steps to nurture his *qi* in the long term, he would recover completely. The patient learned a lesson from this brief relapse and after three additional treatments, along with taking better care of his *qi*, he made rapid progress.

"Doctor, What's Wrong with Me?"

Many thousands of people suffer from ill health that takes them to see their family doctors, yet with no firm diagnosis ever made. Symptoms can include frequent colds, sore throats, swollen glands, tiredness by day, broken sleep by night, headaches, lack of concentration, depressed mood, dizziness, dry or watery eyes, stiffness of joints, aches and pains, heavy limbs, weakness, and unsettled tummy. The list is a long one.

When such patients attend a TCM consultation, they usually report that the family doctor couldn't really say what was the matter with them. Not infrequently blood tests come back normal and antibiotics and painkillers are ineffective. Such conditions are often put down to a postviral reaction, or to stress. Sometimes antidepressants are tried in case the bodily symptoms are due to depression.

Many patients end up wondering if they are making a fuss about nothing and become reluctant to bother the doctor. They know something is not as it should be, although they can't say exactly what it is. Sometimes this chronic state of poor health progresses to ME. The diagnosis is often finally made only reluctantly after many months or sometimes years, on the basis of having excluded other causes rather than because the syndrome is recognized in its own right. By now the patient may well be suffering from other problems such as candida (thrush) from the repeated use of antibiotics, or from side effects from the continued use of painkillers.

The importance of maintaining a strong *qi* has already been emphasized. Now we will look more closely at how the body's immune system works and how the level of *qi* directly influences the immune response.

Consider what happens when someone gets a common cold. This is often blamed on the bad luck of catching a virus. You hear people say "So-and-so gave me their cold!" In TCM, we use the term "pathogenic *qi*," which can be thought of as an enemy army attacking you. In the same way, in the West we talk about bacteria and viruses getting into the body. **The crucial point is that *qi* only becomes pathogenic (harmful) when body-*qi* is already weakened.**

Healthy *qi* is like having your own army that can ward off potential invasion. It activates the immune response, which counterattacks with white blood cells (often showing up as an increase in the white-cell count). When the battle is fierce, there is a fever due directly to a rise in the body's *yang qi*. The battlefield is strewn with casualties, and secretions (mucus, discharges, or diarrhea, depending on where the battle took place) carry off the dead and wounded. These are all signs of the inflammatory response, which shows that the body has the strength to fight back.

If the blood is checked as soon the fight is over, everything appears to be back to normal. You might conclude that despite feeling a bit drained, it's time to go straight back to work. But from the TCM point of view, a normal blood picture can be seriously misleading. What has happened is that nearly all your "soldiers" are dead. Those remaining have been posted on the frontier (in the bloodstream) but there is no internal protection, for the body-*qi* has all been used up. In TCM, this is known as *qi* and blood deficiency.

In China, it is customary for a person getting over a cold to stay home and rest a few more days before going out. This gives time for *qi* levels to rise and restore the immune system. During this time, if we are attuned to our bodies, we will sense the need to get extra sleep. Unfortunately, the modern work ethic often drives people straight back to the office. And even if we do stay home, our minds are liable to be busy with everything there is to be done. **We need to be aware that mental activity alone can block the recovery of body-*qi*.**

What are the consequences of returning to work prematurely? The enemy forces (pathogenic *qi*) soon find a way back in. Because the defenses are down, the territory is overrun. Lacking the soldiers to stand and fight back, there may not even be any signs of infection. Yet the patient can't shake off the feeling of being unwell, and various symptoms start cropping up.

The correct use of antibiotics can be lifesaving, but they work best when the body can still fight back and use the extra ammunition. When the problem is one of *qi* deficiency, repeated use of antibiotics often makes the problem worse because they eradicate the normal bacteria of the intestine, leaving the way open for more harmful bacteria or fungal infections like candida to cause further problems.

A hundred years ago, physicians relied more on nature for recovery, and taking rest was understood to be important. The approach now widely taught in medical schools is largely one of intervention with drugs, and the value of rest is not generally taken into account.

TCM continues to regard rest as an essential aspect of treatment because of the need to strengthen *qi*. When the *qi* is strong, there is no question of blaming someone for "giving you his or her cold." Your body knows just how to protect you, provided you have been giving it the care and attention it deserves!

A Hysterectomy Avoided

A fifty-two-year-old hospital administrator came to the clinic asking for advice. She was worried that she would lose her job because her capacity to carry out her duties was going downhill. The problem was one of heavy menstrual periods over the past year, during which time she had felt exhausted, with sweating, hot flashes, restless sleep, and palpitations during exertion. Her gynecologist recommended that she have a hysterectomy. She was sure she did not want a hysterectomy if it could be avoided, but neither did she want to lose her job.

On TCM examination her *qi* was found to be very weak. Her tongue was large and pale, indicating *yang* deficiency, in this case resulting from overwork and worsened by her blood loss. But there were also signs of *yin* deficiency, such as cracking joints, sweating, poor sleep, and restlessness. Since she never took a lunch break, her baby *yin* had been neglected and the problem had become a vicious circle.

Treatment consisted of acupuncture, during which the patient went into a state of deep relaxation, and a prescribed daily course of Chinese herbs. One week later, she reported that her strength was returning and there had been fewer palpitations. After the second treatment, not only did the heavy bleeding stop but also her periods ceased entirely. Now that her *qi* had been corrected, instead of requiring a surgical menopause, nature had stepped in. Encouraged by feeling so much better, she began practicing *qigong* daily. One year later she remains well, enjoys her work, and travels widely, including to the Far East.

Joints Cracking—*Yin* Lacking!

A twenty-nine-year-old osteopath came to the surgery complaining that his joints had unaccountably begun clicking during movement. There was no pain and he had a full range of movement, but being a specialist in joints, he was puzzled and slightly worried. He had also experienced tiredness for some weeks.

TCM examination of the tongue showed evidence of early *yin* loss, with less than normal coating and a small crack on the tongue. When questioned, the patient admitted that lately he had been thirstier than usual. When asked if he took a lunch rest, he said that because he had recently been so busy seeing patients, he had begun working nonstop through the day. He was treated with gentle acupressure and told he must take a one-hour lunch break and make sure that after eating he could lie down and rest undisturbed. One week later, his symptoms were completely gone.

This case of early *yin* deficiency was easily corrected. The patient was young and when he realized the importance of nourishing baby *yin* by resting during a proper lunch break, he immediately rearranged his schedule.

The combined effect of overactivity and neglect of baby *yin* leads to a characteristic syndrome. In the early stages, people feel good, find themselves moving fast and talking fast, even feeling a bit "high." Body and mind have gone into overdrive, but the joints, like a machine overheating, are running dry. *Yin* maintains the lubrication of the joints, which is essential if they are to last a lifetime. The danger here is that if *yin* deficiency is left untreated, in time irreversible arthritis can occur.

What the Back Can Tell Us about Q*i*

More working days are lost due to back injuries than any other form of illness. Back problems have reached epidemic proportions, yet in the West treatment is often limited to bed rest, painkillers, or major surgery.

A young musician attended the clinic, having suffered severe back pain for four days. It had come on acutely when he was bending over; since then he had not been able to stand up straight.

TCM examination showed that the coating of his tongue was patchy (the "map" tongue of severe *yin* deficiency), indicating damage in the kidney and stomach areas. Acupuncture was given to the region of the lower *dantian*. After a few minutes, the patient stood up without pain. The doctor then questioned him on his diet and warned him against staying up late at night. The young man confessed to loving hot Indian food, going to bed late, and sleeping late in the morning.

How did the doctor know about the patient's lifestyle without asking? The visible damage to the kidney and stomach areas on the tongue told its own story.

Strong kidney *qi* is very important for a strong back. It is like the seed from which a plant grows, a life force welling up in the kidney meridian from the sole of the foot, passing along the lower spine on its way to the kidney and other internal organs, and continuing up to the tongue. Just as a healthy plant keeps producing yet more seeds, kidney *qi* is continually revitalized by all the internal organs of the body. The fundamental nature of kidney *qi* nourishes all body processes and gives rise to the sexual urge, at its height in the young adult. Kidney *qi* needs to be conserved with care. If it is squandered through overactivity or misuse, be it mental, physical, or sexual, the time will surely come when the back gives way.

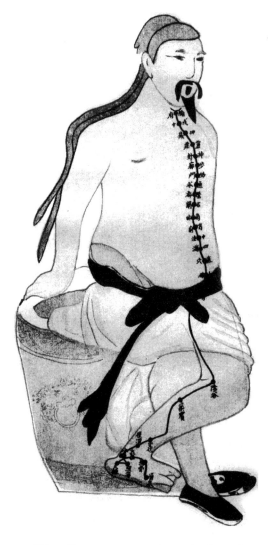

Kidney Meridian

The Chinese routinely soak their feet every night in hot water to nourish the source of kidney *qi* as it wells up from the soles of the feet; they also wash their buttocks in warm water to assist the upward flow of the *qi*. (Other aspects of maintenance of kidney *qi* will be covered in the section on daily health care.)

Chronic disturbances of *qi* in any of the internal organs will show up in the back, either as pain or as local tenderness if acupressure is applied (the "positive reaction"). **This is because the back is a hologram for the whole body.** The pathway of the bladder me-

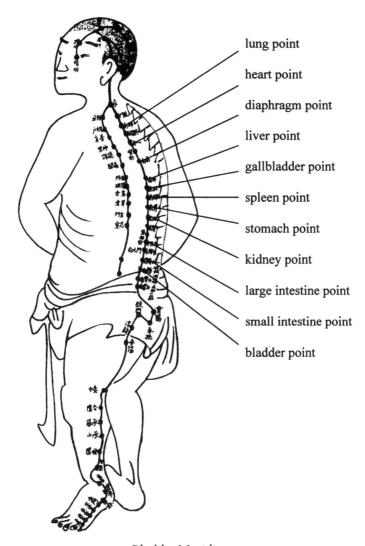

Bladder Meridian

ridian illustrates this clearly. Emotional problems and grief (affecting heart *qi* and lung *qi*) can cause upper back pain, while problems arising from the abdominal organs show up in the middle back and pelvic organs in the lower back.

In the case of the young musician, his back problem had just occurred for the first time. As a young adult, his back should have been strong and supple, and for mechanical weakness to develop, his *qi* must have already been damaged for some considerable time.

If he continues his previous lifestyle, he will risk his back symptoms becoming chronic. However, if he heeds the information-*qi* his back is giving him and makes the necessary adjustments to his lifestyle, he will fully recover. The hot curry and spicy food he eats at night have been burning up liquid *yin* needed for the maintenance of kidney *qi*, so he must give them up.

Many TCM patients seek relief from back pain radiating to the hip, which is often diagnosed as sciatica caused by a slipped disc. Closer examination may reveal the presence of other symptoms, including migraine, emotional distress, neck and shoulder pain, and stiffness and tenderness below the ribs. These symptoms are typical of an imbalance of *qi* in the gallbladder meridian, as discussed previously.

Some patients seek TCM for back problems only after conventional medical treatments, including surgery, have failed to help. Fortunately, acupuncture can be effective even where there is scarring as a result of surgery.

The TCM Approach to Multiple Sclerosis

Western research on multiple sclerosis has concentrated on how nerve cells become inflamed, resulting in weakness and loss of sensation that can affect any part of the body. The only treatment that has been shown to work is betaferon, a new drug that reduces the frequency of relapse in some patients. This is, of course, an important discovery. But western medicine has yet to find the cause of the disease.

TCM documentation of this illness and its origins first appeared twenty-five hundred years ago in *The Yellow Emperor's Canon of Medicine*. Since that time treatment has been aimed at both prevention and cure. The following case study illustrates in some detail how the disease can arise, how it is diagnosed, and how treatment is carried out.

A thirty-five-year-old accountant came to the clinic with a six-month history of progressive weakness and heaviness of the limbs and numbness from the waist down. She had recently been diagnosed as having MS and was still in shock at the news.

On TCM examination, her lower *dantian* was found to be weak and the level of her "sea of *qi*" was very low. The body of her tongue was bright red. The stomach area of the tongue had a midline crack and a yellow coating that extended to the kidney area (see page 9), indicating stomach and kidney "heat" caused by a rise in *yang*. This *yang* reaction is a sign that the body is reacting to pathogenic *qi*. But in this case, the redness of the tongue and the cracking in the stomach area of the tongue also demonstrated a serious, underlying deficiency of *yin*. This is what had allowed the pathogenic *qi* to attack in the first place.

As is frequently found in MS, the stomach meridian was indeed weak. This meridian is essential for the distribution of *qi* and blood, and its weakness was contributing to the underlying deficiency of *yin*. The kidney meridian also was painful on acupressure, suggesting a urinary problem. The patient admitted she had been suffering from a urinary infection since just before the onset of MS symptoms and this had continued on and off ever since.

It became clear with a review of her history that the patient had become *yin* deficient due to years of an overactive lifestyle. Both her stomach meridian and kidney *qi* had been affected, making her vulnerable to the urinary infection.

In TCM, kidney *qi* nourishes the bone marrow, which in turn nourishes both the blood and the brain. This is the final link in the chain of causation in this patient's illness. Nerve cells are very delicate and need constant nourishment by healthy blood. Without strong bone marrow, the nervous system is severely affected. An analogy can be made to the root system of a tree, which draws up moisture and nutrients from the soil.

During the first acupuncture treatment, the patient reported a strong tingling sensation down both legs. By the third treatment, she remarked that her limbs were feeling stronger and lighter, and her urinary infection had begun to clear. After five treatments, normal sensation and power had returned. As to the future, it was explained to her that from now on, she must slow down and conserve her *qi*.

The rapid response in this case was possible because the illness was treated in its early stage. Where symptoms have been present for many years, however, the nerve damage may be extensive and much longer treatment is required to alleviate symptons.

If this case was studied from the western medical viewpoint, the first question asked would be, "If this illness was triggered by a urinary infection, why doesn't everyone suffering from urinary infections get MS?" Such a question would miss what is fundamental to TCM. **Every patient is a unique, sensitive network of interacting life processes, so each individual case must be looked at afresh.**

Consider a plant, previously healthy but now with its leaves dying back. As every gardener knows, dying leaves can be the common end point of many disorders. The problem may lie with soil that is too dry or wet, too acid or alkali, lacking in nutrients or over-rich. The root system may not have had room to expand because the soil was too compacted. The plant may have been infected with fungus or other microorganisms, which is especially likely to happen if it wasn't strong and thriving in the first place.

Any of these problems can result in leaves dying back. So it is with MS, which in TCM is considered to represent the end point of a variety of underlying disorders. The task of the clinician is to identify the particular causation at work in each individual patient. Factors that can play a part include improper diet, lung infections, acute trauma, and overexertion. We will briefly consider these in turn.

The healthy stomach meridian can cope with the absorption of all kinds of foods, but when *qi* is low it is not strong enough to handle the digestion of rich foods. Just as overfeeding a plant will cause it to wilt, overeating will result in weakness and heaviness of the limbs. This is why the stomach meridian will need treatment, along with a light nonfatty diet.

The lungs are responsible for the circulation of body fluids *(yin)* that nourish all the meridians. With pneumonia and respiratory infections in general, the heat of the inflammatory reaction exhausts the fluids, much as the soil around the roots of a plant may dry out. The supply of moisture to the nerve cells then fails. In cases of physical injury, the balance of *qi* is profoundly upset. Getting back to normal requires the same remedy as for a plant blown over in a storm. An uprooted plant will perish unless care is taken

Stomach Meridian

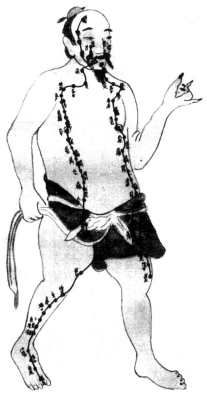

to set it back in the earth and tie it to a support while it regains its strength. As for overexertion, many MS sufferers believe that weakness must be combated with strenuous exercise. The fallacy here can be compared to the assumption that all plants are hardy, when many varieties, some of which produce the finest blooms, need warm and sheltered conditions to grow successfully.

In every case, treatment of MS is directed at increasing the *qi* and blood flow to the nerves and muscles, but this is effective only when the underlying problem has first been correctly identified.

A Child with Asthma: No Need for Steroids

A three-year-old boy who had suffered from eczema and asthma since infancy was brought to the clinic by his parents. The asthma had steadily worsened. He was now using inhalers and taking frequent courses of steroids, which greatly worried his parents, for long-term steroid use can cause permanent damage. The child lacked energy, his appetite was very poor, and his sleep was disturbed. The family had been told by the hospital specialist that there was no other treatment.

On examination, the little boy's tongue was dark red, with no coating in the stomach, kidney, and lung areas of the tongue, indicating severe *yin* deficiency. He was pale, drawn, and extremely listless.

Treatment by acupressure and *qigong* was given, which took about ten minutes. The little boy lay on his back, cooperating very well and showing no fear. By the end of treatment, the coating of his tongue had returned to normal, indicating that his *yin* deficiency had already been corrected, and the color had returned to his face. His breathing had also improved. His parents were told that he would not need steroids and he should return the following week for a further treatment.

The doctor left the room to attend to another patient. A few minutes later the little boy rushed into the reception area followed by his amazed parents. He was shouting out that he was hungry and wanted chicken. For months his parents had been coaxing him to eat, with little success. They asked whether it was all right to give him chicken. The doctor reassured them, explaining that because the stomach *qi* was stronger now, his appetite had corrected itself.

The next week, the parents reported that the boy had needed no steroids, was sleeping and eating well, and was asthma free. With a big smile, the mother added that before coming back to the clinic, her son was saying he was going back to see the magic doctor! A second gentle treatment was given to help the child maintain the new balance of *qi*, and at the time of writing, one year later, he has remained well.

This case illustrates that from the TCM point of view, it does not matter if a condition has been present for years. Provided the imbalance of *qi* can be corrected, the result will be good.

Why has asthma become so common? In the view of TCM, two risk factors are combined. First, in western cultures, a baby may not be encouraged to ventilate and stretch its lungs by normal crying. Instead, a pacifier is stuck in its mouth because the parent feels so overprotective that the child is never allowed to cry. This can result in a weakness of the lungs. A second factor is the influence of parents who are either unduly anxious or tense, or who themselves have a health problem. This results in a weakening of the parents' *qi*, putting the child at further risk.

To explain this more fully, we need to understand how environment-*qi* flows from person to person. *Qi* always flows from a higher level to a lower level, just as water always flows downhill. The child grows up in the environment of the parents' *qi* and depends on the quality of that *qi*, just as a sapling needs moisture, warmth, and sunshine to grow into a strong, young tree. When the parent's *qi* is low, the child's *qi* is weakened, its *dantian* will be underdeveloped, and it will be highly vulnerable to pathogenic *qi*, including germs and pollution. In the case of asthma and eczema, the problem arises specifically from weakness of the lower *dantian*. The lower *dantian* vitalizes kidney *qi*, and strong kidney *qi* is required to nourish the lung. In turn, the lung nourishes the skin, so it is not surprising that asthma and eczema frequently occur together.

As if this were not enough, there is the further danger of the child's *qi* draining to the parent when the energy-*qi* of the parent is very low. Just when it most needs protection, the child becomes even more vulnerable. This underlines that when an individual is sick, the environment-*qi* must always be taken into account. The next case study highlights this point.

Who Is the Patient, Mother or Baby?

A young woman came to the clinic asking for help with her one-month-old baby. Ever since birth, he had been fretful and crying, unable to settle and sleep properly. The baby had been examined medically and there was no apparent cause for this problem.

On questioning, it turned out that the mother had been seriously ill during the last part of the pregnancy. Before and during the birth she had suffered from high blood pressure (preeclamptic toxemia). Once the baby was born, the mother started feeling better. The baby, though, did not thrive.

On TCM examination, the baby was crying and weak, evidently exhausted, and could not be consoled by the worried mother. His face was tinged blue-gray. The doctor held the baby and patted its spine from the top downward. The baby jerked twice and then exhaled deeply. His body relaxed instantly and his face became pink. At once he fell asleep.

Then the doctor turned to the mother and inspected her tongue, which was dark red with orange coloration around the edge, showing stagnation and toxicity. All her major meridians were abnormal, as indicated by the "positive reaction." Acupressure and acupuncture were given accordingly and the condition of her *qi* improved, though it could not be fully restored to normal at this first visit.

As soon as the baby was handed back to his mother, he began crying again. She was advised that until her next visit she should get help with looking after the baby while her own condition improved. One week later she returned. Grandma had been helping care for the baby, who had been much easier to manage. After the mother's *qi* was given further treatment, the baby was placed in his mother's arms, and this time he happily cuddled up to her, to her great delight. There were no further problems with the baby.

This case illustrates three points. First, the cause of the problem was not in the baby but in the mother, even though the problem had presented itself in the baby. This is not uncommon, for babies are highly sensitive to the parents' *qi*. This mother had been ill with toxemia and from the TCM point of view her *qi* was still stagnant and toxic, which had affected the baby. Only when the mother's *qi* was back to normal could the baby enjoy being close to her.

Second, the baby needed help in cleansing himself of the accumulation of his mother's *qi*. The jerking when his spine was patted was a sign that *qi* was being mobilized; he was then able to release the toxic *qi* by breathing it out. His sensitivity to his mother's *qi* was evident when he became distressed on being returned to her before she had fully recovered.

Last, it should be noted that the baby was expressing a disturbance of *qi* of which the mother was not aware. This is because human beings do not function as closed systems but, rather, at the

tempted to quench their thirst with alcoholic drinks. Since alcohol is "heating," still more *yin* is burned up.

No wonder people sometimes come back from vacation drained of both *yin* and *yang*! Their bodies have been going flat out, trying to adjust to the new demands being made on them while away on holiday. Once back home, the old problems soon surface again.

> A thirty-six-year-old woman experienced headaches, sweats, thirst, broken sleep, and fatigue. She was diagnosed *yin* deficient and was making good progress with treatment. Then she unexpectedly disappeared for a couple of weeks. It was winter, and when she returned she explained that she had treated herself to a relaxing holiday in the tropics. She had spent two weeks basking in the sun beside the sea, expecting to feel wonderful. The only problem was that her headaches had returned, her sleep remained poor, and she continued to feel tired. When she came back home, she had to admit that she felt worse than when she went.

Why should this be so? *Yin* provides the body with coolness and calmness, so going to a hot climate and soaking up the sun when you are *yin* deficient is doing more harm than good. This is especially true of winter vacations, because the level of *qi* follows the seasons. During winter, *qi* runs deep and the body is "closed down." Flying off to a hot climate makes a sudden demand on the body, which responds by bringing the *qi* to the surface. A body that is healthy and resilient can cope with the change, but for people who are already deficient in *yin*, further loss of *yin qi* through sweating and overheating in the sun only makes matters worse.

What is it that makes holidays such a source of stress? Often the tension rises even before the holiday begins. People are so anxious to make sure they are going to have a good time that getting away can be more like a military operation than a chance to unwind. Deadlines have to be met before closing the office, clothing and accessories need to be bought, and there is all the worry about taking everything that might be needed, so that by the time the longed-for destination is reached, everyone is exhausted.

Finally you have arrived and the serious relaxing can begin. No more rushing about, no telephones to answer, nothing to do except enjoy yourself! This is a dangerous moment because out of the blue comes a splitting headache, or a heavy cold or sore throat, or you find yourself aching all over with sheer fatigue.

These symptoms are especially common in people who live highly organized and tightly structured lives and who don't have the time or inclination to listen to their information-*qi*. Such people tend to force the pace, rather like central government pushing on at all costs with its own program instead of being prepared to take the voice of local government into account. The body is calling out, but nobody is listening!

Not surprisingly, the moment the controls are removed and there is a chance to relax, the body makes itself heard. What the body is saying is that all is far from well. Nor is a holiday break going to compensate for a life of high-level stress.

Rather than getting annoyed by this noisy protest by the body, it is better to take notice and listen to the communication. Unwelcome though the symptoms are, understanding what your body is telling you could make this a turning point in life. Are you really happy with how your life is going? Is it just a matter of changing the pace, or is it something more? What steps do you need to take to live in harmony with yourself? Your inner voice can tell you, provided you stop and listen.

PART THREE

Learning to Trust the Wisdom of Your Body

Mind and Body in Harmony

The five colors blind the eye.
The five tones deafen the ear.
The five flavors dull the taste.
Racing and hunting madden the mind.
Precious things lead one astray.

Therefore the sage is guided by what he feels
and not by what he sees.
He lets go of that and chooses this.

—Laozi, *Daodejing*

WHEN WE CONTEMPLATE the world of nature around us, we find a deep truth in everything we observe. **There is always a good reason for how things are!** At first glance, this might seem obvious. Yet a lot of human suffering arises because we believe we know better than nature.

Mankind has made some wonderful discoveries in science and medicine. The trouble arises when we try to rule nature instead of remembering that we are part of nature, right down to the chemistry of every living cell. In her wisdom, nature has arranged for each cell to function as a miniature universe, with millions of atoms vibrating in balance and harmony. Chemical transmitters called neuropeptides flow from cell to cell, comprising an information system designed by nature to promote and sustain physical and mental well-being.

This information system has been studied in recent years by biophysicists using the concept of "coherency." Coherency can be compared to an orchestra playing a symphony. All the individual

musicians have their own parts to play, but only when they play together is the sound of the symphony created as the composer intended it to be heard.

Similarly, the DNA in the nucleus of every living cell encodes
the same kind of information system that first breathed life into
matter. Our many different types of cells know just what part they
each need to play. **This coherency will take place naturally if only
we don't interfere with it**. An orchestra needs a well-designed concert hall, with warmth and light and a quiet, receptive space in
which the music can be heard without interruption. Similarly, the
body needs a calm and serene mind, like the quiet of the concert
hall. If the doors of the concert hall are thrown open, however, or
people start getting to their feet, talking, and interrupting the music, the orchestra will soon be in difficulties. Likewise, mental agitation and stress will disturb the harmonious workings of the body.

**Ancient wisdom tells us that when the mind is peaceful and
body-*qi* is flowing freely, we live happy, long, and healthy lives.
This is the true art of relaxation, the cornerstone of the Daoist
way of life going back five thousand years.**

The calm mind is alert but tranquil. It is at one with the body and
because it follows the rhythms of nature, it is at ease with the way
things are. What does this mean in practice? The first step is to learn
to relax. Then we can take a fresh look at the whole picture of life
instead of just looking through one pair of glasses, the ones sitting on
our own noses! We see that many problems exist only because we
make judgments about how things ought to be and expect things to
be the way we want them to be. This is not the way of nature.

It is worth clearing up a point of confusion that has existed ever
since the *Dao* was first introduced to the West. An early error of
translation led to the use of the term "Tao," a word widely used to
this day. In Mandarin Chinese, *"tao"* means "cover over," which has
a very different meaning from that of *Dao*. In everyday usage, *"Dao"*
means "the Way." **In its deeper meaning, even in Chinese, *Dao* cannot be defined in words, for it expresses a totality beyond words.**

Relaxed Mind, Relaxed Body

Empty yourself of everything.
Let the mind rest at peace.
The ten thousand things rise and fall
   while the Self watches their return.
They grow and flourish and then return to the source.
Returning to the source is stillness, which is the way of nature.

—Laozi, *Daodejing*

RELAXING MEANS slowing down. First and foremost, it means slowing down the mind. **Only when the mind is calm does body-*qi* start to flow in accordance with nature's rhythm.**

Qi normally flows at about twenty centimeters a second. When you see someone practicing *taiji* (Tai Chi), the movements appear to be in slow motion, rather like a person sleepwalking. The reason is that they are timed to the flow of *qi*, which allows the practitioner to concentrate the *qi* and harness it to strengthen the body.

Relaxation is the first stage of *qigong*. With instruction and regular practice, we can become sensitive to the movement of body-*qi*. Since *qi* is the essence of all creation, this awareness takes us straight to the heart of the cosmos where there is perfect balance and harmony. Being truly at one with nature leads to a feeling of deep joy and happiness. Since this knowledge has been gathered over thousands of years, it is worth seeing how it compares with some recent scientific findings on the human subject.

A recent experiment demonstrated that during normal sleep

71

the total body intake of oxygen slows down until, after six hours of sleep, the rate has fallen by 8 percent. In contrast, a study of *qigong* practitioners in deep relaxation showed that after just fifteen minutes, total oxygen consumption fell by 16 percent. When less oxygen is needed, body rhythms have a chance to settle down and synchronize. The aging process itself slows down, which is why *qigong* masters are notoriously long-lived. In the natural world we see this, for instance, with turtles. Their low metabolic rate allows some species to live for up to two hundred years; thus in China the turtle is an ancient symbol of longevity.

Another area of research concerns brain-wave patterns. EEG studies show that when our eyes are open, the whole of the brain is electrically active, and there is no single dominant rhythm. When our eyes are closed, a synchronized wave of electrical activity pulses at nine to twelve cycles per second. This is called the alpha rhythm, and it is strongest at the back of the brain. (This rhythm pulses at the same speed as the earth's natural electromagnetic field, a phenomenon known as Schumann Resonance.)

Qigong practitioners have been shown to produce the alpha rhythm also in the front and top regions of the brain and with a voltage five times greater than normal. This state of brain activity when the mind is deeply relaxed is associated with a number of important findings.

In everyday life, many people put up with cold extremities, unaware that this is a telltale sign of underlying tension or stress. It has been shown that relaxation causes the circulation of blood to improve so that not only do hands and feet stay pleasantly warm but the flow of blood to the internal organs is also improved.

States of stress and anxiety cause the level of lactic acid in blood to rise. Research carried out on *qigong* practitioners shows a level of lactic acid four times lower than in calm but untrained subjects.

Another measure of stress is illustrated by the galvanic skin response, which is the basis of the lie detector test. Lying under questioning causes a physiological stress reaction that provokes a release of adrenaline (the fight/flight response) causing the capillaries under the skin to constrict, perspiration to increase, and skin temperature to fall. The immediate effect can easily be measured as a lowering of electrical resistance across the skin surface. On the other hand, the more relaxed a person is, the higher will be the skin resistance. Skin resistance normally averages fifty thousand ohms. In one study of *qigong*, the average skin resistance was found to be two hundred thousand ohms, an effect which continued for twenty minutes after the test period, indicating that these subjects were exceptionally calm and relaxed.

Another important indicator of stress is the level of cortisol in the blood. Studies have shown that people who are emotionally overburdened or physically stressed produce high levels of this substance. Cortisol is one of a number of corticosteroids produced by the adrenal glands to enable the body to cope with the stresses of ordinary life, but when the output is too high for too long, the body's immune system becomes suppressed. (Athletes know about this because if they train too intensively, the prolonged stress raises their corticosteroid levels to abnormally high levels and their resistance to infections is weakened, which can result in prolonged viral illnesses.) One study of *qigong* practitioners showed their cortisol levels to be 25 percent lower than the normal population, indicating how much the deeply relaxed mind has a direct effect on the chemistry of the body.

Just how sensitive living creatures are to stress was demonstrated in an experiment on white mice. The mice were placed in a comfortable, stress-free environment, with just one exception. Randomly, and without warning, they were subjected to minor but unpleasant stimuli. Their corticosteroid output rose, eventually resulting in adrenal exhaustion, shrinkage of the thymus gland, and falling T-cell production; in short, their immune systems broke down.

Cancer is the result of abnormal cells multiplying out of control. It is well recognized that a healthy immune system protects against cancer. The abnormal cells are rooted out and destroyed before they have a chance to start growing into tumors. In contrast, normal cells do not multiply out of control because they show "touch inhibition," reflecting their sensitivity to neighboring cells. Research on cyclic AMP (adenosine monophosphate), which is normally produced in small quantities throughout the body, has shown that introducing this substance into cancer cells can restore their sensitivity to touch inhibition. The cyclic AMP carries the information needed to "reprogram" the cancer cell to revert to normal functioning.

Qigong produces a 15 percent increase in the level of cyclic AMP after just thirty minutes. Even more striking, in one study of chronically ill patients being taught qigong and practicing it for three months, an overall rise of 25 percent was found. A further study was carried out with qigong masters "treating" samples of blood in test tubes by holding their hands ten centimeters away for five minutes. Cyclic AMP levels in the blood samples rose by 28 percent.

These studies have been conducted in China under the direction of Professor Xie Huanzhang in Beijing. Another line of research, carried out in Germany by Professors Zhang Changlin and Fritz Popp, has revealed that all living systems radiate photons (the smallest units of light energy) of extremely weak intensity. These particles, called biophotons, are generated continuously within the cells of the body. They travel through the body at the speed of light, and sensitive apparatus can detect them being emitted from the body at about eight hundred biophotons per second.

Qigong practitioners have been shown to radiate very high biophoton levels, as many as forty thousand per second. Current research on the significance of this phenomenon, which physicists call a "chaotic state," challenges us to revise the old model of "mind over matter" in which we think of the mind as exerting control over body processes, much as a conductor leads the orchestra. **What we may be finding out is that the calm mind releases the whole body to "freewheel" so that the pattern of coherence encoded deeply into its fundamental design can take over.** In other words, this orchestra needs no conductor, for the qi of the cosmos plays itself through each and every musician with perfect timing and tuning.

Ancient Medicine:
A Hundred Generations
of Study

Heaven and earth last forever.
Why do heaven and earth last forever?
They are unborn,
So ever living.
The sage stays behind, thus he is ahead.
He is detached, thus at one with all.
Through selfless action, he attains fulfilment.

—Laozi, *Daodejing*

WE CAN NOW SEE just how much TCM accurately forecasts what modern science is demonstrating in the laboratory. **The fundamental principle can be summed up as follows: avoiding emotional stress gives peace of mind. Peaceful mind strengthens body-*qi*. Strong *qi* protects the organs of the body against pathogenic *qi*, ensuring health and natural longevity.**

In the ancient Daoist medical tradition, we are warned of the converse principle, with an image of terrible destruction from within. The person who shirks moderation and instead indulges in emotional excess falls victim to greed, jealousy, and stupidity. It is said that within the body three worms begin to grow. Too much mental strain causes a worm inside the head to start growing; too much emotional turmoil feeds a worm in the chest; and vanity, lust, and greed give rise to a worm in the stomach region. Unless the

75

situation is corrected, these three worms will rot the body from within!

This powerful image of internal corruption is not confined to Daoist texts, as shown by a dream recently reported by a patient seeking advice for migraines and fatigue. The TCM diagnosis was spleen deficiency caused by mental exhaustion and chronic anxiety. After acupuncture, the patient was able to relax and look calmly for the first time at the problems facing him and his wife. To his great relief, they were able to talk together constructively. Then he dreamed that he was picking at his body and pulling worms out from under the skin. When he described the dream at the next TCM consultation, he was reassured that the dream was a sign of progress. His symptoms had gone and so had his spleen deficiency.

It has already been noted that pathogenic environment-qi can attack the body if body-qi is already weak. The danger comes from outside, and according to TCM the invasion first has to penetrate the skin, then the muscles and the meridians. The internal organs are affected when pathogenic qi enters the meridians and is carried deep into the body. But the danger is greater still when the disturbance of qi arises from within, which is why we now need to consider the part played by emotions in causing illness.

According to TCM, excessive emotions, especially when they are dammed up, act directly and immediately on the internal organs. There is no filter to damp down their impact on the body, which can take place without any conscious awareness of the harm that is going on. The five internal organs are linked with the emotions as follows:

- liver — anger
- lung — grief
- heart — unbearable joy
- kidney — sudden fear
- spleen — worry

Any excessive emotion will target the related organ. The mechanisms by which the internal organs are affected can be complex, but to single out just one, let us look at how anger damages the liver.

When anger is sparked off, there is an immediate surge of *qi* that brings a rush of blood to the head. This leaves the liver drained of blood, seriously depleting it of *yin* and causing immediate damage to the organ. To avoid this, from the TCM perspective it is best to have attained a state of mind in which all situations can be faced without anger. Failing this, if anger should be kindled, it must be acknowledged, for if suppressed, the *qi* is left churning around in the stomach and chest regions. All the meridians are liable to be affected by this turmoil as the *qi* tries to find a way out. For example, the natural flow of the gallbladder meridian, which runs from the head down to the feet, can be thrown into reverse by the agitation of *qi*, resulting in a severe headache or even a migraine.

Daoist sages teach that anger can damage *yin* but also that excessive joy can damage *yang*. A balance is required which calls for moderation in all things. Too much of any one thought, emotion, or action will disturb the circulation of the *qi* and blood of both *yin* and *yang* and their regulation will suffer accordingly. The effects can be summarized as follows:

- Excess anger, through its effect on the liver, upsets the *qi* and the blood of the whole body.

- Excess grief, through its action on the lung, causes pain in the region of the chest, respiratory illnesses, and skin disorders.

- Excess joy weakens heart *yang qi*, causing heart disease.

- Excess fear harms kidney *qi*, with the result that willpower is drained, the spine is weakened, and the bowels, urinary system, and sexual organs are affected.

- Excess worry exhausts heart and spleen *qi* with resulting lack of energy and concentration.

- Excess thinking causes loss of mental clarity.

- Excess talk wastes your *qi* and leaves you feeling worn out.

- Excess dwelling on the past, especially nostalgia, drains vitality.

- Excess rushing about wears down the physical body.

- Excess criticism of others makes you become sour in both temperament and appearance.

- Excess leisure dissipates the will.

- Excess attachment to any one thing becomes an addiction.

- Excess desire, including too much sex, results in mental turmoil and spiritual decline.

As the *taiji* makes clear, too much of any one thing leads to an imbalance which goes against nature. Ancient wisdom tells us that if instead we curb excesses, we experience all the beauty and richness of life revealed in the eternal play of *yin* and *yang*. The daily round is one of infinite variety and discovery when we are masters, not slaves, of the world of the five senses. Peace of mind and a healthy body are the two most precious assets in which we can invest.

The Art of Knowing Your *Qi*

See simplicity in the complicated.
Achieve greatness in little things.

In the universe the difficult things are done as if they are easy.
In the universe great acts are made up of small deeds.
The sage does not attempt anything very big,
And thus achieves greatness.

    —Laozi, *Daodejing*

WHEN **YIN AND YANG** are in balance and the *qi* is strong, we sleep deeply and wake refreshed. The body feels light and ready for action and there is a natural desire to get up and start the day. As the body instinctively responds to our needs, our activities flow with spontaneity and creativity. Mind and body are working as one.

When *yin* and *yang* are not balanced, mind and body cannot work together. For example, you wake but your eyes don't want to open. You tell yourself to get out of bed but your body wants to stay behind and you have to drag it along with you by an effort of will. By the time you have had a cup of coffee, you feel ready for action. But later, when you take a break, you find you can't relax. You want to read the paper but your eyes feel strained and start watering. You reach for a cup of tea but accidentally knock it over. You decide to go for a walk but as soon as you get up your legs start aching and you change your mind. At night, instead of drifting off to sleep, you toss and turn as you become acutely aware of your body processes. You find your heart is beating heavily, or your breathing seems tight, or you feel hungry and have to get up to have a snack. You are definitely out of sorts with your body!

How is it that we can get so far removed from the natural unity of mind and body that evolution gave us over hundreds of thousands of years? The answer is very simple. We are in such a rush that we have forgotten how to stop and listen to what the body is trying to tell us for our own good. To find out more, the first step is to create the calm that is so lacking in our modern world.

When the mind is calm and the body at rest, the sensitivity of the body information system increases dramatically. Take, for example, minor earth tremors, which in the Far East are quite common. If you are moving around, you may not notice anything going on. If you are sitting quietly at the time, you feel the house sway and notice the lamp swinging, causing you to feel momentarily dizzy. More familiar to the western world might be the sensation of sitting quietly in a garden and suddenly becoming aware of the breeze rustling the leaves of the trees. In this relaxed state, small signals from around us that would ordinarily be overlooked are amplified and readily noticed.

This heightened awareness applies equally to signals coming from within the body. At a subtle level, the body is always in motion. Digestive juices are being secreted, hormones are circulating, qi is flowing; indeed every minute, thousands of cells are dying and thousands more are newly created. The body is engaged ceaselessly in a dynamic process of adjustment and adaptation, all aimed at keeping a balance in which mind and body can work effortlessly as one. Without giving it a moment's thought, we are benefiting from the nonstop work the body is doing on our behalf. When we are hungry we eat, when thirsty we drink, when tired we sleep, when cold we put on warm clothes. The information system is taking care of us and protecting us from harm around the clock.

The feedback that the information system of the body gives us comes in a variety of ways and can be categorized as either whole body reactions or specific body reactions.

Whole Body Reactions

To tune in to our reactions, we have to set aside our logical, rational selves and be open to intuitions and sensations that we might otherwise be tempted to dismiss.

Before taking any course of action it is first necessary to consult your body and see how it feels about what you are doing. Suppose you have arranged to go to a meeting. On that day you find yourself reluctant to go. Your information-*qi* is giving you signals of discomfort, perhaps heaviness or weariness, and the energy just isn't there. The western approach is to tell yourself you have made the commitment so you must attend. The alternative is to ring up and make your apologies. The problem most people in western society immediately encounter is guilt. This has to be faced. There will be occasions when your own body-*qi* must come first, something we are not accustomed to heeding.

Looking a bit further into the kind of warning your information system is giving you, we see that there can be more than one meaning. It may simply be that you do not really need to attend this meeting although at the time it seemed necessary. It could be that your body is not well or that you are tired, and the message is saying that you cannot afford to go because your *qi* is weak. You don't want to let your colleagues down, but if your *qi* is weak and you do go, you will not be doing them any favors. Either your fatigue will make you poor company or you will be forced to make a big effort to be bright and communicative. Unfortunately your underlying deficiency of *qi* will affect your colleagues just the same, leaving them unaccountably weary. Remember that *qi* flows along an energy gradient from high to low so that their *qi* is bound to be drained by you. In the end, the effort you made will have further depleted your own *qi*.

At a deeper level still, the information-*qi* serves to warn you directly that a particular event is best avoided or could even be dangerous for you. Qi can travel like radio waves from person to person and place to place and is able to operate beyond the bounds of space and time.

A choir of twelve children were due to meet at a local church one evening. For a variety of reasons, on the night in question none of them was able to go. One missed the train, another got ill, a third scorched her blouse, and so on. That same evening there was a fire in the church, which was completely destroyed. Without realizing it, everybody had by one means or another found ways to protect themselves from harm.

Another example concerns a couple that was coming home late at night after going to the opera. They reached the place where they normally turned left to take the road home, but at that moment the man, who was driving, just couldn't turn the wheel. Instead he found himself carrying straight on to where the road ended at the beach. He was so surprised at what had happened that he turned the car around and very cautiously and slowly made his way back. Two and a half miles down the turning to their home they came upon the scene of a road accident in which a car had brought down a power line across the road. If they had been driving as usual, they would have crashed.

There are many similar examples in the literature on extrasensory perception. A person may even have a vivid premonition of disaster. But it is important to recognize that when the body sends out a warning, it may be at odds with what the mind is bent on doing. Only later does it become clear what the warning was about. **Often such a warning comes out of the blue. It seems that the sensitivity to such messages is greatest when, far from being worried about anything, one is in a relaxed frame of mind.**

Specific Body Reactions

Each day when you are washing your face, take a moment to check in the mirror whether you have dark rings under your eyes. Are the whites of your eyes clear, or are they bloodshot? Now look closely at your hands. Is the skin soft and smooth or is it rough and dry? Inspect your nails. Is the surface smooth or are there ridges running the length of the nail? Does any part of your body look or feel abnormal—for example, red, swollen, or discolored, unduly hot or cold, tender or painful, itchy or coming out in a rash, numb or oversensitive to touch?

Here the information-*qi* is speaking through the part rather than the whole, in accordance with the body functioning as a hologram as described earlier. All that is required is to stay calm and take notice of what you have observed. Even though you may not be aware of exactly what is wrong, there is no need to become anxious provided you trust your body to get back on track with the right kind of help.

Both whole and specific body reactions reveal an imbalance of *qi*. The problem for most people leading busy lives is that these body reactions pass unnoticed, with the result that the underlying problems accumulate and in time result in serious disorders. If we decide instead to listen to our bodies, there are two steps to be taken. First, we need to pay attention to the communication. In the case of the whole body reaction, this means trusting our intuition at the body level. With the specific body reaction, it means taking the trouble to notice the small but telltale signs that all is not well. Second, in order to read the message accurately and efficiently, we have to stop and relax in order to sensitize ourselves to the underlying imbalance of *qi*.

Assessing the State of Your Health

For the sake of simplicity, three states will be considered in turn.

State One: The healthy person, whose *yin* and *yang* are well balanced and whose *qi* is strong, remains calm in all situations, including emergencies. He does not pay attention to the trivia of life or to events that do not concern him. Yet his concentration on information that is relevant to him is both total and effortless, and he deals with the tasks at hand accurately and highly efficiently. Being free from any sense of urgency, he neither wastes time nor acts in haste. He is never slave to emotions so in daily life he does not get nervous or excited, and even in exceptional circumstances, he is overwhelmed by neither joy nor grief. He is not interested in talking for its own sake, but when he does speak it is measured, concise, and to the point.

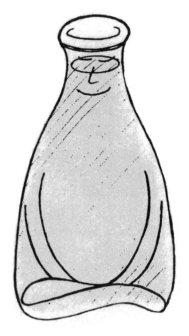

People with these qualities can mistakenly be thought of as somewhat "dumb" because they don't show much response to the external stimuli that excite or agitate many people. Yet when they do take action, they are quietly decisive and don't make mistakes. Because they assess situations calmly

Full bottle of wine

and objectively, the way is open to new and creative insights arising from a deep intuition of what needs to be done and how best to do it. **We can compare this state with a full bottle of wine. Shake it and there is no sound, for since it is full, the wine cannot splash around inside.**

Because the *qi* is full, such people are unlikely to fall ill. Their bodies know what is beneficial to them, and the right foods, the right people, and the right environment naturally attract them. Conversely, they know how to avoid what is not good for them. If they do start feeling unwell, their sensitivity is such that without delay they take the appropriate action to restore their balance.

State Two: *Yin* and *Yang* are out of balance. This person can be completely unaware that there is anything wrong. Yet careful observation of his behavior reveals the underlying problem. Such a person is inclined to be very active, taking on one job after another. He tends to talk a lot and talk fast. His movements, too, are fast, but lack of coordination may lead him to be clumsy. He is liable to

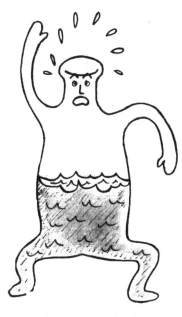

Half-empty Bottle of Wine

be forgetful—going shopping and then not remembering what was on the list, mislaying keys, documents, and the like.

Subjectively, he may feel very alert, even "high," but he can't relax because his mind is always running on ahead. Even when physical exhaustion sets in, he can't "switch off" from what is going on around him because he is oversensitive to external events, no matter how trivial. This results in his rushing around a great deal but not completing tasks or actually getting a lot done.

This condition arises when the *qi* is weakened due to the buildup of emotional or physical stress. In this overstimulated state, there is too much reactivity to the world around, coupled with a loss of sensitivity to the internal needs of the body. Only after such a person is able to calm down does a wave of exhaustion sweep over him. **We can compare being in this state of overdrive to shaking a bottle of wine that is half empty. Less wine means more noise!**

If this state of imbalance is recognized and steps are taken to put it right, the treatment couldn't be simpler. It means slowing down and deliberately creating the opportunity for rest and sleep, including a lunchtime break and a bedtime of no later than eleven o'clock. Both mind and body may take some time to calm down while the *qi* is being restored. During this period of rest, some symptoms may appear that until then had not been able to surface. Rather than taking any medicines, it is best to wait and see if the symptoms subside. If not, they may need treatment with TCM. But essentially, given a little patience and perseverance, *qi* will be replenished, *yin* and *yang* will come back into balance, and the wine bottle will fill right up!

On the other hand, unless remedial steps are taken to correct the imbalance, the condition will get worse, because the person feels energetic and capable and so isn't inclined to stop. There are endless jobs to be done because in this state everything seems urgent, and it is no longer possible to stand back and see the wood for the trees. The underlying lack of *qi* adds to the feeling of pressure; more mistakes are made due to a loss of efficiency and tasks take longer to complete. If the person does allow himself a bit of a break, far from feeling refreshed, he feels more tired than ever and may find himself afflicted with the breakthrough of underlying symptoms. As discussed in the section on holiday syndromes, just taking a couple of weeks off is not going to put matters right.

State Three: The balance of *yin* and *yang* in the human body has deteriorated to such a degree that the information system has been severely damaged. Neither mind nor body can continue to react appropriately to stimuli, whether internal or external, large or small. This is the eventual and inevitable outcome of state two left untreated. Unfortunately, if the person has relied on painkillers, or has been subjected to other drug treatments or surgery that has failed, additional trauma to the information system may have knocked it completely out of action.

The serious depletion of *qi* leaves the person mentally and physically exhausted, yet unable to calm down and recuperate. He is restless, irritable, and in need of sleep but suffering from insomnia. Messages from the body are often contradictory. When trying to sit still, hands and feet may want to move as if of their own accord. When getting up from a chair, the body reacts by becoming so heavy and tired it is almost impossible to move. Pains can start up in any part of the body and the hands and feet may feel numb.

There are two patterns of response to these alarming symptoms, depending on the individual's natural degree of sensitivity. Sensitive people, being highly reactive, soon get overloaded by anything going on around them. Unable to switch off from continuing internal and external stimulation, they become anxious and fearful. Other people's *qi* is so much stronger than their own that the person feels swamped, like a boat thrown about in rough water. Even casual conversation produces intense weariness.

People with less sensitive natures respond somewhat differently. Rather than continuing to react, the system shuts down. As a result, such people don't talk a lot or even complain much. **At first glance, this might look like State One, in which the bottle of wine is full, for in both cases there is no splashing around of wine when giving the bottle a shake. Here, though, it is because the bottle is well and truly empty!**

Closer inspection reveals the difference between the two states. Far from being well, the person has

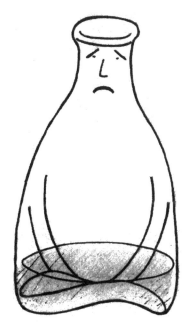

Empty Bottle of Wine

to use what *qi* is left for basic survival. The color is unhealthy, with cheeks abnormally pale or dark. Even severe infections may fail to produce a temperature because the body cannot mount an inflammatory response. There is a risk of hypothermia and the person becomes cold, often beginning with the feet and working upward. It is a dangerous state to be in, for fatal illness can strike with little or no warning.

This state of crisis can be a turning point, however. First, what is needed is accurate and effective expert treatment. With treatment, the *qi* will begin to recover, along with the body's information system. It is also necessary to recognize that the way of life needs fundamental change if recovery is to be long lasting. Indeed, it is no coincidence that many *qigong* masters suffered life-threatening illnesses that inspired them to make a study of *qi* and how to harness it. **With sound advice, guidance, and a determination to exchange old, harmful patterns of behavior for new, health-giving ones, it is possible not only to recover but also to attain a state of health and strength far greater than before.**

Protecting Your Q*i*

The advice that follows is deceptively simple, yet if you follow it, your life will be transformed.

- When you are about to carry out a task, first take a moment to relax. Sit down and close your eyes. Next, gently release your breath in one long exhalation and let your body flop. Now become aware of your whole body. How does it feel? Because you have relaxed, you will become more sensitive to your *qi*. If your body wants to get moving, fine. But if it wants to pause and rest, give it a little of your time.

- Leave gaps between daily tasks. Ensure that you have breaks in your schedule so you don't have to rush from one thing to the next.

- Allow yourself to doze off if you feel like it. This indicates that you have been able to stay calm and not get caught up in the pressures you are under. No matter how busy you are, this will stop you from worrying. Worry does not help you make decisions or work to the best of your ability. Highly creative people maintain the capacity to rest and play even while they are at work.

- Give yourself one day a week when you don't have to follow any schedule. On this day, make your goal to follow what your body asks you to do.

- Every morning and before you go to bed at night, take a minute to observe the condition of your body. Look at your face, hands, and feet. Check for any specific body reactions but also use the opportunity to center yourself in your body. Close your eyes and sense what your whole body feels.

- When you feel that body and mind are not working well, don't push yourself. Change your plans instead to suit what feels comfortable and manageable. Reschedule your appointments if necessary.

All this adds up to one thing: the art of learning how to relax and rest. If your body is not entirely well, you need to switch off from all those customary sights and sounds such as the television, radio, and telephone, and especially the conversation which fills up so much of the day. Make yourself comfortable, lie down, close your eyes, and sleep until you wake naturally. Your body will get on with righting itself and, if the problem is not too serious, you will wake refreshed and feeling well again without the need for any tablets or medical attention. If resting deeply doesn't bring about an improvement, then it is time to seek expert help.

Remember that our bodies are not all of a type but highly individual. Some people are by nature sensitive while others are less so. A health problem will show up early in the sensitive type but the response to rest or treatment will be equally rapid. In contrast, while less-sensitive individuals are not so likely to fall ill in the first place, when they do, even a small sign that something is wrong could have serious implications. This is why continuing maintenance of the body is so important. People understand that their cars need regular attention. Similarly, we need to give time and attention to the needs of the body.

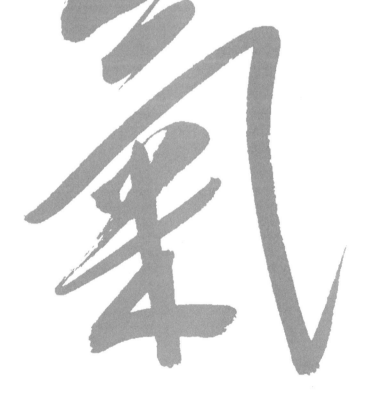

PART FOUR

The Daily Care of Your Body

The Biorhythms of
Yin and *Yang*

> *Knowing others is wisdom,*
> *Knowing the self is enlightenment.*
> *Mastering others requires force,*
> *Mastering the self needs strength.*

> —Laozi, *Daodejing*

THE ANCIENT WISDOM of Chinese medicine teaches that better than any treatment is to avoid falling ill in the first place. There is an old Chinese saying that needing treatment is like beginning to dig a well when you feel thirsty!

To stay fit and live long, it is important to keep in mind how the *qi* of the cosmos influences the *qi* of *yin* and *yang* in the human body. The biorhythms of body-*qi* reflect the cycles of the year, the season, the month, and the day, all of which are determined by the motion of the heavenly bodies.

The *taiji* of the seasons illustrates the cycle of the whole year. You can see at a glance how *yin* and *yang* reflect the changing seasons. In spring, when nature gives birth, *yang* grows and reaches its peak at midsummer. Throughout the autumn it declines, and by midwinter it is at rest until emerging again the following spring. *Yin*, being the mirror to *yang*, grows throughout the autumn and by midwinter is at its peak, subsiding through the spring. In this way, the four seasons flow one after the other, from the warmth of spring to the heat of summer, the cool of autumn, and the chill of winter.

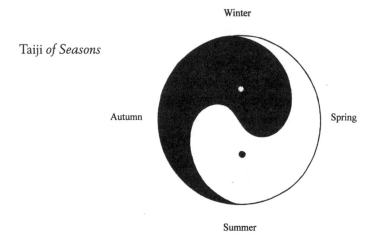

Taiji *of Seasons*

The *yang qi* of the human body is like a miniature sun, radiating outwards and driving away pathogenic *qi*. During the day, it flows over the surface of the body, regulating the opening and closing of the pores of the skin. We saw in Part One how *yang qi* increases during the morning and is at its most powerful by noon, after which it gradually declines throughout the remainder of the day. Any vigorous physical exertion in the late afternoon or evening will make a demand on *yang qi* at a time when it needs to be able to withdraw into the body undisturbed. It is particularly important not to engage in strenuous outdoor activities when the sun is setting. The worst possible time to go jogging is after work. Not only is *yang qi* being burned up when it is already low, but sweating forces open the pores of the skin, breaching a natural defense against pathogenic *qi*.

When a person is too active mentally or physically, the flow of *yang qi* will increase in response to the need. The rise in *yang qi* is possible because there is a reserve of *yin qi* on which to draw. *Yang qi* is like a plant that responds to the heat of the sun with rapid growth so long as its root system can draw up the moisture it needs. But if the growth spurt outstrips the root system's capacity to absorb moisture, the plant wilts. This is the danger for someone living too much on *yang qi*. As with the plant, when the supply of *yin qi* has been used up, life will come to a premature end.

Yin deficiency is one of the most common syndromes encountered in TCM in the west, giving rise to a whole range of problems from arthritis to disorders of sight and hearing and other neurological conditions. Drinking more water is not the answer, for the underlying balance of *yin qi* to *yang qi* needs to be restored.

In contrast to the active nature of *yang qi*, *yin qi* is quiet and calm, governing the internal fluids of the body. It is the female principle and needs to be cherished and protected by *yang qi*, which stands firm like a warrior guarding the door of the household. This is the key to the true harmony of *yin* and *yang*.

Yin qi is nourished in two ways. First, a daily rest at lunchtime will help the birth of baby *yin*. This allows *yin* to grow steadily throughout the afternoon and reach its strongest at midnight. Second, since *yin* is produced from the intake of food, what and when to eat and drink requires special consideration. But the ancient texts warn against two indulgences in particular to maintain good health: Do not overeat in the evening, for each time you do so, it reduces life expectancy by one day. Similarly, avoid getting drunk, for each time it happens, life will be shortened by one whole month.

Safeguarding the biorhythms of *yin* and *yang* calls for certain constraints. Staying up one whole day and night without sleep leads to a loss of *qi* that will take at least ten days to recover. Habitual strenuous exercise during the hours of sunset will deplete *yang qi* and endanger future health. Failure to take a rest break between 11 A.M. and 1 P.M. will starve baby *yin*, and staying up late between 11 P.M. and 1 A.M. likewise starves baby *yang*. The ancient texts also make it clear that sex should be avoided during the hours of sunset since this is a time when *yang qi* is on the wane.

The Daoist view of the rhythm of life is that human activities should flow gently like running water. Accordingly, all activities, whether walking, talking, standing, sitting, sleeping, eating, drinking, or exercising the mind, need to be in balance, neither too little nor too much. Then the *qi* will flow easily and harmoniously.

Such considerations may feel like an infringement of personal freedom, and in a world given over to extremes, moderation may seem a dull option. Yet we need to bear in mind that the health-

care advice that follows is all aimed at bringing vitality, health, and happiness to those seeking it. The hundred generations that lived before knew how to cherish and value life. It is our good fortune to be able to reap the harvest of their knowledge and experience.

The Right Way
to Start the Day

THE BEST TIME to wake is with the rising sun, for at this time the body-*qi* is rising too. If you need to empty your bladder, do so right away but then spend a few minutes quietly lying on your back in bed with your eyes closed, and do abdominal breathing (see "The Art of Breathing"). Imagine the sun shining on your body and relax from head to foot, keeping the mind calm and still. Before you get out of bed, have a good stretch and gently massage your face with your hands. Once out of bed, keep warm by putting on your clothes or a dressing gown. Start by cleaning your teeth and washing your face in cold water. The cold water stimulates the circulation of the blood and closes the pores of the skin, helping protect against pathogenic *qi* when you go out.

This is the time for outdoor exercise, weather permitting. If you enjoy jogging, do it now. The strongest *qi* comes not from pushing yourself so that your heart is racing and you are pouring with sweat but doing just enough to feel warm and with the pores of the skin just opening so that you are nearly but not quite sweating. If the sun is out, it should feel as though you are taking a shower in sunlight. If it is not sunny, as your body-*qi* rises you can still experience the warm glow from within. Some people prefer walking. If you practice *qigong* or *taiji* (Tai Chi), face the east because you will immediately benefit from the *yang qi* of the sun, no matter if it is cloudy. Apart from the fresh air, it is good to find somewhere with grass and trees so that you will absorb the environment-*qi* of nature.

Back home, a warm, unhurried, and nourishing breakfast is essential. While you are eating, set aside any worries you might have and concentrate on enjoying the food. Don't talk or read while eating, and if you have the radio on, it is best to listen to gentle, harmonious music. This allows your body to relax and ensures that digestion will proceed smoothly. When breakfast is over, allow yourself enough time to get to work without rushing.

The Art of Breathing

TO BREATHE IΓ TO LIVE. Every newborn baby cries out in order to expand its lungs with air for the first time and continues to breathe until respiration ceases with the ending of life. It follows that we all know how to breathe!

It does not follow that we understand breathing as an art and a skill that can bring us health and longevity. Breathing as an art originated in China and is thought to date back ten thousand years to the New Stone Age. We know from engravings more than five thousand years old that *qigong* was practiced then just as it is now, with the same postures and method of breathing.

The human figure shown on the pot (see page 100) has eyes half closed, the stomach region is expanded with the hands resting on the lower *dantian,* and the legs are apart and flexed as in *qigong* today. The mouth is slightly open as in "turtle" breathing, one of the oldest methods of breathing on record. An ancient text tells the origin of turtle breathing.

A man happened to fall down a disused well and could not climb out. No one came to rescue him and he thought his days were over. His one companion was a large turtle living at the bottom of the well, who seemed in excellent health despite the lack of food. The only thing the man could think of doing was to copy the turtle as it turned its head from side to side, opening its mouth as if gulping down air. He found that not only did his hunger pangs go away but also he

Pot from Quinghai, ca. 4000 BC

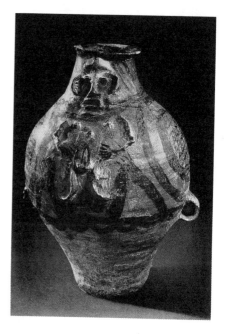

remained fit and well. One hundred days later, he was rescued and his *qi* was found to be stronger than ever!

Breathing correctly is essential to health. Turtle breathing is one of a number of techniques in *qigong*, including fetus breathing, feet breathing, and abdominal breathing, all of which have in common the purpose of replenishing *qi*. The method focused on here is abdominal breathing because it is fundamental to health and easy to make part of everyday life.

First, a few facts. Each lung contains some 1.5 billion air sacs called alveoli. If the lining of all the alveoli could be stretched out flat, it would cover a tennis court! Nature has given us this delicate membrane so that oxygen can be absorbed through it into the bloodstream and the gaseous waste product, carbon dioxide, released when we breathe out. When we breathe shallowly, as happens with chest breathing, we use only one third of this membrane for the exchange of gases. Sitting slumped reduces the proportion to one sixth.

Research has shown that mental activity increases the oxygen intake of the brain by as much as three times the resting level. A combination of shallow breathing and mental exertion, whether one is busy thinking or getting emotionally excited, leaves the brain cells with reduced oxygen. The carbon dioxide level falls, taking the oxygen level down with it (known as the Bohr effect). Compare this with the combination of abdominal breathing and a calm mind; carbon dioxide remains stable at the optimal metabolic level while every brain cell is saturated with oxygen. No wonder your body and mind feel light and happy.

Abdominal breathing stretches the diaphragm. Since nine major meridians pass through the diaphragm, this breathing powerfully stimulates the *qi* and the blood and massages the internal organs. As the diaphragm is lowered, air is drawn right down to the bottom of the lungs and oxygen intake is increased. The technique can be carried out standing, sitting, or lying down.

Let your whole body relax and focus your mind on the lower *dantian*. This is located in the midline, at a point behind the navel and in front of the kidneys. Rest your hands, one lying over the other, over the navel. (Women should place the left hand on top,

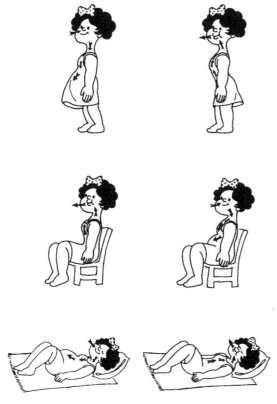

Abdominal Breathing

and men the right. The difference reflects the cultivation of *yin* [right side] for the woman and *yang* [left side] for the man.) Next, breathe out with the mouth slightly open, gently contracting your abdominal muscles while keeping the chest relaxed and still. Feel the stale *qi* being squeezed out from the abdomen and released with the breath. Now close the lips, gently touching the roof of the mouth just behind the front teeth with the tip of the tongue, and keeping your chest still, slowly breathe in through the nose. Imagine the air flowing right down to the lower *dantian*. As the air flows in and the muscles relax, the abdomen will begin to swell. When it is full, pause naturally for as long as it is comfortable, and then gently release the breath through the nostrils until the abdomen has gone down. With each breath, picture fresh, clean *qi* entering the body and the stale *qi* being exhaled. If you hear gurgling noises, it is a sign that the internal massage is going well. Don't try to suppress the gurgles but enjoy them. To begin with, expect to take about six breaths a minute. Later, you may find you are only breathing two or three times a minute.

Everybody, young and old, can benefit from abdominal breathing. Many people never use the diaphragm to breathe, because of stress or simply because of the excitement of living in the fast lane. Underlying bodily tension causes rapid, shallow breathing and a tendency to talk too fast without stopping. Even if a person is otherwise physically well and taking regular exercise, the *qi* in the lower *dantian* can remain dangerously weak because the lower *dantian* never properly fills. This is why people who pride themselves on keeping fit can still be vulnerable to many illnesses, including high blood pressure.

In contrast, people who regularly practice abdominal breathing have excellent circulatory and lung function. Their speech is unhurried and between sentences they breathe naturally from the lower *dantian*. The voice is firm and naturally commands attention. There is always energy on hand because the abdominal breathing is continually renewing *qi*. (Singers know how important it is to breathe from the abdomen because when they go on stage, which would cause most people to shake with nerves, they can stay relaxed and produce a strong, steady voice.)

Many successful people from all walks of life have learned how to use the breath in this way to overcome anxicty and increase their effectiveness in a wide range of situations. Abdominal breathing can also help with quitting smoking. Instead of taking a cigarette, try abdominal breathing.

Abdominal breathing needs to be practiced until it becomes second nature. Make sure that you give it time before you get up in the morning and before going to sleep. You can practice anywhere and at anytime, and the more you do, the better you will feel.

The Rhythm of
the Four Seasons

THE ANCIENT TEXT OF *The Yellow Emperor's Canon of Medicine* sees the rhythm of human life as subject to the seasons, just like the rest of nature. We are advised that throughout the year we should get up at sunrise and go to bed by the time it gets dark. In the temperate zones, this means sleeping much longer in winter than in summer, and the difference becomes greater the farther north and south you go. Since the industrialized world disregards such biorhythms, we are left to decide for ourselves how closely to follow this rhythm of nature.

Spring is the season of growth, when *yang* is rising. The birth of new life is to be seen everywhere as seeds germinate and trees come into leaf. It is best to get up at sunrise and retire to bed when it gets dark. Start the day with a relaxed walk outside, or around the garden. Let your hair hang loose, avoid tight clothing, and feel yourself growing within, for you too are part of nature. Open your heart to the beauty all around you. This is the time of year to be giving birth to your creativity, in whatever form it takes. The weather is changeable, but dress warmly, for the body has been acclimatized to winter and the *yang qi* needs to be protected, otherwise a cold snap will have the same effect on the body as on flowers that blossom too early. When the weather does become milder, lighten your clothing gradually so that there is no abrupt change. Diet, too, needs to harmonize with the season. Spring is the time for "warm," sweet foods like rice, peas, dates, and walnuts, and pungent foods such as peppers, onions, garlic, and ginger that encourage the *yang qi* to start rising.

Summer is the season of nature's prosperity, as the *yin qi* of earth merges with the *yang qi* of heaven. Trees and vegetation are lush and new growth has given way to a glorious display of flowers. Now is the time to get up early to imbibe the *yang qi*. Enjoy the long days and be sure to rest at lunchtime. Then the heart is nourished and you won't be troubled by the heat of the summer. Enjoy the long evenings too, for there is no need to go to bed while it is still light. The beauty of nature acts as an inspiration to remain calm and cheerful while nurturing the *qi* through the long summer days. Take pleasure in outdoor activities. Body-*yang* is strengthened and as perspiration opens the pores of the skin, the *qi* is helped to flow freely. Strenuous activity, on the other hand, should be avoided, for heavy sweating depletes *yin*. For this reason sex too is best avoided during very hot weather.

The body should be protected from any sudden chill such as taking a cold shower, getting cold outdoors, or consuming refrigerated food or drink, because the effect of cold is to block the flow of *yang* in the internal organs. Salty and sour foods such as prawns, seaweed, and soybeans are beneficial because they help prevent *qi* from leaking from the body when the pores are open. Meals should be light and not too fatty since digestion needs *yang qi* and much of the *yang* has moved to the surface of the body during the summer.

Autumn is the season of ripening fruits and crops ready for harvesting. The weather cools and the winds begin to stir. *Yang qi* starts to move inwards, causing the leaves of the trees to change color and fall. Body-*qi* also withdraws, making way for *yin*. Rise with the sun and go to bed early. As the weather becomes harsh there is a danger of emotional turmoil; it is all the more necessary to stay calm and peaceful, for the *qi* needs safeguarding for the winter months ahead.

It is a good time of year to be building up *qi* with regular practice, be it *qigong*, martial arts, or meditation. As the weather cools, change in good time into warm clothing, ensuring feet and legs stay warm. The clothing should be gradually increased to avoid any sudden overheating that would drive the *yang* to the surface. Similarly, avoid pungent foods, which could have the same effect. It is preferable to eat sour foods which retain the *qi*. These include chicken and prawns, potatoes, and fruit such as tomatoes, apples, and kiwi fruit. Other foods such as chrysanthemum wine, pears, sesame seeds, and honey specifically help *yin* to grow.

Winter is the season of rest. *Yin* is dominant now and *yang* has retreated deep inside. The metabolism of all living creatures slows down and some animals slumber in hibernation through the long, dark winter days. Humans too should restrict their activity in order to preserve body *yang*. It is best to go to bed early and not get up before sunrise. The mind should be calm and contained, like a treasured heirloom kept safe from harm.

On stormy and windy days, stay indoors when possible. The body-*qi* needs to be conserved by keeping warm but not hot. Sitting too close to the fire or sweating from taking a hot shower or bath opens the pores of the skin and *yang* is lost. This is also why clothes should not be hung over a radiator or in front of a fire immediately before putting them on. Keeping the feet warm throughout winter is essential in order to nourish kidney *qi*. Don't forget the nightly routine of bathing the feet in hot water just before going to bed. If you do need a hot water bottle, it is best to put it down by the feet.

Winter is a good time for physical exercise such as walking or jogging, which moves the *qi* within the body and prevents stagnation but does not bring *yang* to the surface. Exercise until you are warm but stop before you sweat. Practice of *qigong* is especially valuable. "Warming" foods help maintain *qi* and nourish *yang*. These include cabbage, carrots, red beans, potatoes, cereals, walnuts, and chestnuts. One glass of good quality wine, or a tot of whiskey each day after the evening meal helps the circulation of *yang* within the body and drives out the cold.

Water as Medicine

THE CHINEJE CHARACTER *"huo,"* meaning "life," reflects the profound need of all life forms for water. There are two types of water that need to be considered, body water and environment water. The quality of both is of great importance to health.

Character for "Huo" 活 = 氵 + 舌

Life   =   Water   +   Tongue

Body Water

Eighty-five percent of the human body is water. Water is the basic component of blood, in which the white and red cells are suspended and various salts, proteins, and other compounds essential to life are dissolved. Water is equally important inside the cells of the body where, surrounding the nucleus, it forms the protoplasm, which contains complex structures necessary for the functioning of the cell.

Both western medicine and TCM equally recognize the danger signs of severe dehydration, which causes dry mouth, intense thirst, dry and wrinkled skin, and even loss of consciousness and death. But in TCM, particular attention is paid to the daily water

balance of the body because subtle disturbances of balance that
may not be obvious can lead in time to serious health problems
such as brittle bones and arthritis.

In contrast, when the body water is in balance, the skin is soft and
glowing and the body is strong, supple, and resistant to injury. The
joints are well lubricated so that they function smoothly and without
clicking or other signs of friction. The mouth produces plentiful saliva, like drops of clear, fresh liquid (as you see in healthy babies),
there is no sensation of thirst, and the appetite is well regulated.

Normally we produce between one and two liters of saliva each
day. Tension, anxiety, and depression reduce the flow while relaxation and happiness increase it. In *qigong*, great store is set on saliva,
not just as an indicator of the overall condition of the body but also
as a precious juice that confers longevity. It is considered to be the
natural ginseng of the body, and by using exercises that involve clicking the teeth together sharply, *qigong* practitioners encourage a still
greater flow.

Modern scientific analysis of saliva has shown it to be a remarkable fluid. Not only does it contain a number of enzymes needed for
digestion but also laboratory tests have shown it to promote protein
synthesis, reduce bleeding time, and even inhibit the growth of cancer cells. Further, saliva contains immunoglobulins and other compounds that have an antibacterial effect. One study on *qigong*
practitioners showed that their saliva contained twice the usual level
of immunoglobulins.

The condition of the body water can be determined by inspecting the mouth for saliva. If the saliva is thick and sticky or has an
unhealthy smell, then the body water is not clean and there will be
associated blockages in the circulation of *qi*. Such saliva (as well as
any phlegm from the nose, throat, or chest) should not be swallowed but spat out.

There are a number of ways in which the quality and quantity
of body water can be improved.

- Maintain a calm and peaceful mind. Take a nap at lunchtime,
  practice relaxation, and find the opportunity to listen to soft

and harmonious music. When outdoors, contemplate the beauty of nature. Remember to practice abdominal breathing regularly.

- Avoid unnecessary talking and in general keep your mouth closed. An open mouth dries up saliva. At night, lying on your side reduces the chance of mouth breathing and snoring.

- Physical exertion should be taken during the morning (*yang* time) and even so, heavy sweating should be avoided.

- Drink water or green tea frequently, but in small quantities.

- Eat moist foods (porridge or oatmeal is a suitable and nutritious breakfast food, for example).

- Increase the production of saliva by eating slowly and taking time to chew the food thoroughly.

- Morning and evening (and at other convenient moments), click the teeth together thirty-six times, keeping the mouth closed throughout. Fresh saliva will begin to flow, which should then be swirled around inside the mouth by the tongue before being swallowed.

Environment Water

Our body water is continually replenished by water from external sources at a rate of two to three liters daily, although in hot climates it will be more. In addition to the water we drink, we need to take into account the moisture (water vapor) in the air we breathe and the water that comes into contact with our skin when we wash or from exposure to humidity.

Only unpolluted rainwater and snow are naturally "soft." As groundwater seeps down through the sedimentary rock to the water table, it reacts with minerals in the rocks to form sulphates, chlorides, bicarbonates, and the oxides of calcium and magnesium. An excess of these two oxides causes the water to become "hard," altering its taste and texture. Boiling the water will take away much of this, and ion exchange filters, as are now widely used in the home, also improve the quality. Unfortunately, water is often additionally contaminated with nitrogenous compounds from fertilizers, chlorides from human and animal waste, toxic chemicals from industrial waste, ferric oxide (rust), and chlorine added for sterilizing purposes.

Such water, far from being a medicine, is a chemical cocktail best avoided whenever possible. Boiling and filtration go some way toward purification but better still is to use mineral water that has come from deep springs. Man-made pollution does not penetrate the filtration through the rock formation and the trace minerals present are naturally occurring ones.

The benefits of country air, trees, and especially nearby water have long been recognized in TCM as playing a valuable part in the treatment of a wide range of conditions, including bronchial asthma, essential hypertension (high blood pressure), muscle and joint strains and sprains, arthritis, skin and stomach problems, and coronary artery disease. Practitioners of *qigong* seek trees (especially pines) and water because of the quality of the *qi* that can be detected.

The beneficial effect of trees and water on health has been corroborated by research into the chemistry of anions. Anions form when water molecules naturally split in two, releasing positively charged hydrogen atoms and negatively charged anions. This happens during thunderstorms, in sunlight, over oceans, and by rivers, lakes, and waterfalls. Trees, especially pines, also give off copious quantities of anions as the water drawn up from the ground evaporates from the leaves. (In urban areas there are less than five hundred anions per cubic centimeter of air; in the countryside there are three times as many, and close to water, eight times the concentration.) An increase in the proportion of anions (sometimes called air vitamins) in the atmosphere has been shown to sharpen the senses, invigorate mind and body, increase lung function, reduce blood pressure, improve sleep, accelerate wound healing, and result in increased physical energy and mental well-being. Here is another example of ancient wisdom supported by the findings of modern science.

If you live in a city, make sure that in your spare time you visit your local park, relaxing and benefiting from the moisture of the trees and plants. If there is no park nearby, make sure that you have plenty of fresh air in the house and grow as many house plants as you can.

Now let us return to TCM to see how water can best be taken as medicine in daily life. Such was the attention to detail that two thousand years ago more than forty types of water were identified for medicinal purposes! We will confine ourselves to just a few of them and their uses.

Hot water promotes *yang qi*. Since the *yang qi* of the body rises at breakfast time, cold tap water should be avoided in the morning and instead water that has been boiled should be drunk, warm on its own or as good quality green tea. At any time when *yang qi* is weak, as when the body is cold, warm water again will be beneficial.

There are only two occasions when iced water should be drunk. The first is when the internal heat of the body has become excessive due to hot weather, and the second is to help detoxify the effect of alcohol, also regarded as "heating." Drinking iced water at other times can cause the blood vessels of the stomach to constrict, harming stomach and spleen. At mealtimes especially, the blood supply to the stomach needs to flow freely and iced water is the last thing it needs.

Spring water from mountain streams is cold and clear, dispersing internal heat and alleviating irritation. Well water, which is neutral in character, can also be used, provided it is fresh and clean.

The morning dew is particularly beneficial. Since one of the most common disorders in the West is *yin* deficiency, try starting the day by putting on some old clothes, going into the garden or nearby park, and standing on the grass. Gently practice abdominal breathing with your eyes closed and sense if your body wants to make contact with the grass. If so, lie down on the grass, enjoying the sensation of moisture close to your skin and the smell of the damp ground. Spend a few minutes like this, letting the dampness of the dew be absorbed by the body while continuing abdominal breathing before going back indoors to change your clothes. The *yin qi* you have taken on board will remain with you throughout the day.

Similarly, when the air is damp or drizzly, don't complain about the lack of sun. Instead, take the chance to go for a gentle walk, inhaling the cool and refreshing *yin* in the air. Feel its calming and soothing effect as you breathe it in and draw it down to the lower *dantian*.

Rainwater, being naturally soft, can be collected for making quality tea. Also drink it as a natural remedy for mental agitation and distress, signs of unbalanced *yang qi*. Snow water, too, is soft and pure, good for alcoholic "heat" and inflammation and infections of the eyes. (These two waters are known in China as Heaven Spring water).

Seawater is regarded in TCM as "warm" in nature and therapeutic for a number of skin disorders including itching. Hot sulphur springs are used to treat skin infections as well as inflammatory skin conditions.

Tea drinking, which in the ancient traditions occupies a place of honor, deserves special mention here. The best water for tea should be soft, sweet tasting, and light in texture, as found in snow, spring water, or rainwater. River water and well water are more dependent on local conditions, while bottled mineral water can be selected according to taste. Tap water is never desirable. The *qi* in tap water is destroyed by pollutants and chlorine that react with polyphenols present in the tea leaf, producing oily compounds that float on the surface and giving the tea a bitter taste. If tap water must be used, let it stand for a day so that the chlorine can be released, or better still, use filtration and then let stand.

Fresh green tea is rich in vitamins, with a wide range of trace elements, alkaloids, and amino acids, as well as lipopolysaccharides and sugars. At least two or three cups a day are beneficial, more if you are an active person. Tea will even compensate up to a point for vegetables and fruit if these are in short supply. After eating, wash the mouth out with tea to clean the oral cavity.

The quality of the tea is as important as the quality of the water. The best tea is Dragon Well, highly prized in China and not generally exported. It is said that if you drink this tea made in spring water from West Lake, Hangzhou, you have truly lived life to the full! Of the dozens of varieties of tea in China, a smaller range is available from Chinese supermarkets now established in many urban centers in the West. Try these teas for yourself. Some will be pungent, others fragrant, some invigorating, and others mild and relaxing. Sprinkle some leaves in the bottom of the cup; add boiling water and leave to infuse for a few minutes. The leaves will usually float and then settle. Any remaining leaves on the surface can be gently blown out of the way before sipping.

Green tea is "cool" in nature and good to drink in spring, summer, and autumn, and when the body is hot. Chrysanthemum tea is best for dispersing body heat in very warm weather. In winter, black tea of the kind that most people in the West drink with milk is "warming," and may be preferred.

To make sure the body absorbs the water and its nutrients to the best effect, it is important to be in a peaceful and unhurried frame of mind when drinking tea. Don't wait until you are thirsty and then gulp it down. The Chinese speak of "sampling" tea, first enjoying the smell and then sipping it a little at a time. When the cup is finished, simply pour on fresh hot water. The flavor from the leaves will improve with the second cup, and good quality leaves will often last the whole day, the tea becoming suitably light by the evening.

Tea cleans the mouth of phlegm, the unpleasant mucus that collects when body water is dirty and stagnant. It directly detoxifies and cleanses the stagnant body water so that the breath becomes sweet smelling, and it promotes the digestion of fatty foods. Nature has been truly bountiful in providing us with a medicine that tastes so good and gives so much pleasure!

Washing Is a Skill!

WASHING IS NOT JUST a matter of cleaning the skin. As explained in Part One, the skin is much more than the body's covering, for it is intimately related to the meridians. The pores of the skin not only open and close on account of sweating but at a subtle level they also regulate the flow of *qi*. It is helpful to remember this when you wash and care for your skin.

When you get up in the morning, wash your face with cold water. Better still, take a cold shower. This brings several benefits. It directly stimulates the elastin in the skin to contract, reducing bagginess and wrinkles and helping to maintain a glowing, youthful complexion. The pores of the skin close, preventing bacteria from entering that may cause spots and skin infections. Likewise, the body is protected against pathogenic *qi* when you go outside, especially when it is cold and windy. Cold water also stimulates the circulatory and nervous systems and activates the immune system.

This approach runs counter to modern cultures in which hot showers or baths are frequently taken in the morning, often including washing the hair. This is not desirable, for since the morning is *yang* time, the heat causes the body to lose *yang qi* just when it is being built up for tackling the tasks of the day ahead. Another drawback is that the heat brings the blood to the surface of the body, and it is then unavailable to the stomach and bowel for digestion of breakfast.

We can see how easily a harmful chain of events arises. If baby *yang* has not been nourished during the night, we wake still tired and reluctant to get up. To console ourselves, we linger in a nice, warm bath, with the unfortunate result that more *yang qi* comes to the surface and is lost from the body. Then we rush to get breakfast in time. We eat hurriedly while hearing about the latest bad news on the radio, further disturbing body-*qi*. Finally we are off into the cold with pores wide open, often traveling to work in crowded situations where pathogenic *qi* abounds. By midmorning *yang qi* is running low, so we keep going on caffeine, burning up what little *yang qi* remains. No wonder so many people suffer from indigestion, catch colds, and battle weariness all day long.

How often should we wash the whole body? This will depend, of course, on how active one is and on the work one is doing. It also depends on whether, through the right daily actions, we have been taking good care of body-*qi* (ensuring that the breath is clean and fresh and the body keeps a pleasant smell). Under these circumstances, it may be enough to bathe or shower only once or twice a week. On other days wash just the face and neck, using cold water in the morning and warm water at night. (Cold water is stimulating and may interfere with sleep.) Wash the armpits, the genitals, and buttocks in warm water, not forgetting to soak the feet in hot water before going to bed and giving them a gentle massage at the same time.

If you do feel like a warm bath or shower after a long and tiring day, have a light snack first, since low blood sugar combining with the blood and *qi* rising to the surface of the body can cause faintness and weakness. Don't eat too much, because the blood and *qi* needed internally to aid digestion will be in short supply. The bath or shower should be taken well before bedtime, and the water should be pleasantly warm but not so hot that you start sweating, which will cause a loss of *qi*. When you wash your hair, dry it thoroughly straight away

Nourishing Kidney Qi

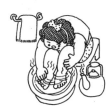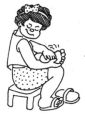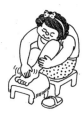

and above all, don't go to bed with it still damp or expose yourself to a chill, for if the meridians on the scalp are affected, it can result in headaches and dizziness, impair your hearing, and even cause hair loss. Wrap up well as soon as you get out and avoid draughts in order to protect the body from any chill.

After the bath or shower, drink a little boiled water to replace moisture lost from the skin and have something light to eat to replace leakage of *qi*. Since washing your hair can drain heart *qi*, a snack will protect you from night sweats or disturbing dreams.

The therapeutic effect of the shower or bath is to open and cleanse the pores and stimulate the circulation of the blood and *qi* so that the stale *qi* of the day can be dispersed, the bacteria on the skin washed away, and body and mind helped to relax in preparation for sleep.

Saunas are not advisable for people in poor health, but when the *qi* is strong they are beneficial. If you take a sauna, make sure it is a time of relaxation, for nothing burns *yang qi* faster than an overactive mind. As the temperature rises and the pores open, *qi* flows freely to the surface and leaves the body with the sweat. When water is poured over the fire or hot rocks, the humidity becomes saturated and the *qi* is reabsorbed into the body through the skin, mouth, and lungs. The effect is a cycling of *qi*, which is cleansed as it circulates. Next, when you plunge into the cold pool or shower, the pores instantly close down because of the sudden temperature change and because you are still deeply relaxed, the blood vessels and nerves react in a split second to the new situation. This is a safe but powerful training exercise for the circulatory and autonomic nervous systems.

Last, there is what *qigong* practitioners call air baths, sun baths, moon baths, and forest baths. These baths don't need water, for you can bathe directly in *qi!* When taking an air bath, it is best to stand with the feet parallel and apart, the width of your shoulders. Next close your eyes. Bend the knees slightly and imagine that your buttocks are resting on the edge of a high stool with your weight evenly distributed on your feet. Gently bring your lips together, the tip of the tongue touching the roof of the mouth behind the front teeth. Let your arms hang down by your side, palms forward, slightly away from the body so that air can circulate under the arms.

Now picture yourself standing between earth and sky, suspended from the heavens with
your feet held by the earth so
that your spine is being gently
stretched. Become aware of the
vast expanse and depth of the
cosmos all around you. Spend a
minute or two gently practicing
abdominal breathing. Now visualize all the pores of your skin
opening like a thousand windows, so that the fresh *qi* of the
cosmos flows into your body.
You may feel yourself becoming
light, warm, or having tingling
sensations. If so, you are simply
experiencing the flow of *qi*.

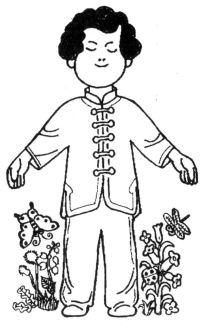

Air Bath

Maintain this for about ten minutes, then have a good stretch, hands
clasped above your head, and open your eyes. The immune system
will be strengthened, the central nervous system vitalized by the absorption of ions, and all metabolic processes stimulated by the re-
plenishment of *qi*.

The sun bath is a regular part of *qigong* practice. It should be
taken in the morning during *yang* time and is best done at sunrise and
when wearing loose clothing. Prepare as for the air bath, with the
same posture and facing the sun with your eyes closed. (If it is
cloudy, face where the sun would be.) This time, picture opening a
thousand windows to the light of the sun as it pours into you. You
may notice after a while that it is getting very bright behind your
closed eyelids, and on a cloudy day it may seem to you that the sun
has started shining. It can be a surprise to open your eyes and find it
is still just as cloudy outside! What has happened is that the *yang qi*
of the sun has lighted you up from within.

Natural light is composed of colors of many different wavelengths mixing together to produce "white" light. The many

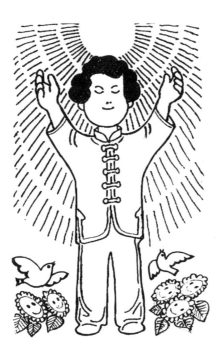

Sun Bath

beneficial effects of taking a sun bath are due to this wide range of frequencies of light being absorbed by the body, from infrared through all the colors of the rainbow to ultraviolet. Sunlight is anti-bacterial, anti-inflammatory, and antiallergenic. It irradiates the skin, converting sterols formed by food products to vitamin D, which is essential for bone formation. It regulates the production of melatonin by the pineal gland, now recognized to govern a whole range of hormonal biorhythms. TCM holds that these beneficial effects, including the immune response, result from the strengthening of *yang qi*.

As a health warning we should note that the sun bath is not to be confused with the recreational pursuit of sunbathing. Prolonged exposure to the sun has been shown to cause premature aging of the skin and increases the likelihood of skin cancer.

When taking a moon bath, first let the moonlight pour in through your eyes. Then gently close them, while continuing to visualize the moon and absorbing its *qi*. Let the cool light trickle down to the middle *dantian* and experience the silvery light shining within the middle *dantian*, expanding to fill the whole body from within. Moon bathing will strengthen body *yin*, helping you to remain calm and

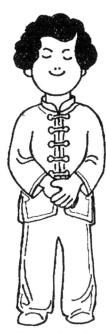

Qigong *Standing Posture after Bathing*

serene at all times, and will promote deep and restful sleep. To sound one note of caution, as we have remarked earlier, an excess of either *yin* or *yang* will turn into its opposite. This is why at full moon *yin qi* can become an activating force (indeed, some people find it hard to sleep on those nights), so bathing too long in the light of the full moon may leave you wide awake.

Last, there is the forest bath. While walking among trees or in a forest, relax and open yourself to the nourishing *yin qi* given off by the trees. Let it bathe you from head to foot. You may experience a smell of perfume as you absorb the *qi*. Try standing by different trees. You may find you can sense a variation in the strength and quality of the *qi* that allows you to select the place of your choice. According to *qigong,* young, healthy trees will cleanse and freshen your *qi*. For strengthening your *qi*, choose a strong and mature tree. (In China, *qigong* practitioners give the same regard to trees as to human beings. Ancient trees such as pines or ginkgoes, both of which can grow to more than a thousand years old, are not used for their *qi*. Instead such a tree is honored with the greatest respect.) Forest baths are good for producing deep relaxation and happiness, cleansing and strengthening body-*qi*, and vitalizing the heart, lungs, and immune system.

How to Dress

CHOO**/**ING **WHAT CLOTHE/** to put on when we get up
gives us the opportunity to harmonize with our *qi*, for colors
have a special place in healing, strengthening the internal organs and promoting the flow of *qi* in the meridians. White light is
made up of a mixture of wavelengths, but when the wavelengths are
scattered, as with a prism or a rainbow, we see the different frequencies as bands of color, with red at the short end of the visible
spectrum through to violet at the long end. What makes a piece of
material blue, for example, is that this particular piece of cloth absorbs all the frequencies of light except the blue wave band, which
is reflected back. White clothing reflects all the frequencies while
black is black because it absorbs them all.

In TCM, certain colors, each with its own specific vibration, are
matched with the internal organs (and their associated emotions) as
follows:

- green — liver — anger
- white — lung — grief
- red or pink — heart— elation and great joy
- black — kidney — sudden fear
- yellow or brown — spleen — worry

When you let yourself be guided by your *qi* in deciding what to
wear, you will automatically choose the clothes to suit the internal

condition of your body. If possible allow your hand to move un-thinkingly to the color it selects for you; trust that your body has the wisdom to pick out what it needs. This sounds easy enough, but it takes some practice because we are in the habit of stopping and thinking about what to put on. Alternatively, be sure to take what-ever color feels most comfortable and enjoyable to wear.

When you allow your body to choose for you, by checking the correlation of the color with the internal organ, you can identify the underlying condition of your *qi*. Suppose, for example, you have been feeling irritated. Without giving it any thought, you may find yourself selecting something green. Green is the color for the liver, which in TCM is linked with anger. The green you put on will bal-ance the disturbance of liver *qi* and help to calm you so that you overcome your annoyance.

There are some interesting cultural differences regarding colors and their associations. For many societies, black is the traditional color of mourning. According to TCM, this would be appropriate enough, since grief drains kidney *qi*, which black will help to strengthen. In China, however, white is worn at funerals, because the lung is associated with grief and so white, the color for the lung, will help to relieve the pain of sorrow.

People whose *qi* is unbalanced by excessive thinking will benefit from wearing brown or yellow. Excessive thinking can harm the spleen, which is balanced by these colors.

Red is linked with the heart as a fiery *yang* organ and is the color to wear when you find yourself becoming too elated or overexcited, for it exerts a balancing effect, as in homeopathy where "like is treated with like." Pink has similar properties and is useful where there is a degree of agitation or nervousness. Children are attracted to colorful clothes because their bodies are undergoing many shifts of energy due to the growth of internal organs. Wearing bright and varied colors balances this process and promotes growth and integra-tion, but when they need to calm down, children often instinctively choose pink because it helps them feel more balanced. Not all col-ors—blue for example—are associated with the internal organs.

During the last twenty years, research in China has led to the development of numerical *qigong* in which the information system of the body is linked with ten colors and the ten cardinal numbers:

1. Light blue — balance between *yin* and *yang* — harmonious functioning of body organs
2. Light red — *qi* as a subtle, quivering vibration — calming agitation and overexcitement
3. Grass green — fine-tuning of balance of *qi* — stabilizing and calming heart and lung
4. Brown (and earth colors) — strong surges of *qi* — vitalizing body reactions
5. Light yellow — slow rhythmic oscillations of *qi* — sedative effect
6. Dark yellow — alternating fast and slow waves of *qi* — alerting and arousing effect
7. Dark green — saw-toothed waves of *qi* — motivating and energizing
8. Purple — uninterrupted flow of information-*qi* — enhancing the total human potential
9. Dark red — vertically rising waves of *qi* — transformation and healing
10. Clear yellow — free flow of *qi* in the meridians — balance and well-being

Apart from the color, when choosing clothes avoid tight-fitting garments that can cause stagnation of blood and *qi*. As a general guide, clothing should be soft, loose fitting, and comfortable, encouraging the free circulation of blood and *yang qi*. Clothing should be neither too warm nor too light. As the seasons change, adjustments to clothing should be introduced gradually to help maintain an even body temperature.

At all times, the feet need to be dry, clean, and warm, and when traveling, be sure to take plenty of socks with you, thick and thin, so that you are never caught out by the climate. Likewise, keep the legs warm. In the chapter on "The Flow of Qi in Nature," it was explained that it is better to have the head cool and the lower half of the body warm in order to avoid the "volcano effect" (see "Live Now, Pay Later"). When the lower limbs are colder than the upper limbs, arthritis can set in due to the cooling of the *yang qi* as it rises from the feet.

If you sweat, don't allow the body to get chilled and don't cool down by exposing the body to the wind, for the open pores make you vulnerable to pathogenic *qi*. Wait instead until the sweating has stopped and then change into fresh, dry clothes. If you have none available, take a towel and dry yourself down under the clothing you already have on. In winter, the art is to preserve *yang qi*. As explained in "The Rhythm of the Four Seasons," clothes that have just been heated in front of a fire or on a radiator can cause a loss of *qi* and should not be worn.

Once you understand the principle of balancing and maintaining your *qi*, what to wear becomes a matter of common sense. **If your *qi* is strong, you need not waste energy on worrying about the latest fashion, for nothing is more attractive than a person who is glowing with health and vitality.**

Eating Wisely, Eating Well

TO EAT OR NOT to eat? That is, so often, the question. Common sense tells us we should eat when we are hungry. Yet people who are under stress or whose metabolism is seriously out of tune may experience hunger most of the day, and sometimes during the night as well. This is not something that simply eating more will put right. From the TCM perspective, body-*qi* has got so out of balance that information-*qi* is no longer able to do its job. In this situation, so-called greed is really misplaced need. In contrast, when the *qi* is strong and balanced, then hunger as information-*qi* is highly accurate and sensitive and helps us to establish and maintain a healthy eating pattern.

Yang qi is required for the proper digestion of food, which is why all meals ideally should be taken during daylight hours. In winter, it is best not to have the evening meal later than half past six or seven o'clock, because *yin qi* is now becoming dominant. If you do eat at a late hour, the demand on *yang qi* when it is already low stimulates *yin qi* to burn up, resulting in *yin* deficiency, often with broken sleep, thirst, sweating, palpitations, and restlessness.

A general rule is that you should leave the table feeling that you could comfortably eat a third as much again. This ensures that the stomach is not overloaded and that the toxins produced as by-products of digestion will be safely and easily dispersed. A common problem is that when the *qi* is low, a person is so hungry to start with that the food is wolfed down, resulting in acute bloating and discomfort (one of the reasons why people suffering from bulimia make themselves vomit) and causing subsequent indigestion. Many disease processes are associated with overeating and obesity, including high blood pressure, diabetes, cholesterol and lipid disorders, and heart disease. Eating in moderation helps the *qi* to flow smoothly and regulates the body metabolism. Nature will then prevent these disorders from developing in the first place.

Giving care and attention to how we eat would seem of obvious importance, since eating is fundamental to all life. Unfortunately, the trend in the modern world towards fast food, TV dinners, and precooked meals suggests we have more important things to do than take time to eat as nature intended. From the TCM perspective, this is a big mistake.

As noted in "The Right Way to Start the Day," a warm, unhurried, and nourishing breakfast is essential. This should be at around 7 A.M. but may be later in winter. Certain guidelines apply to all meals; they should be taken sitting down, with sufficient time to relax and enjoy the food. Any disturbing environment-*qi* such as news on the radio or television (the bulk of which is given over to crises of one sort or another) should be avoided. Try eating in silence. If you find it strange to begin with, it probably means that like most people you have become habituated to nonstop background stimulation, and it will take time to adjust. A happy compromise is to listen to music that is calm and yet inspiring. When eating in company or with family, conversation should be light and occasional only. Save more serious discussion for later, for your attention should be given over to enjoying the taste and texture of the food. Children naturally concentrate on what they are eating and can easily be discouraged from chattering if they are set the right example by adults. This approach does not mean that meals need be boring or gloomy; on the contrary, people can come together companionably, relishing the food and sharing harmonious environment-*qi*.

While we are eating, much of the blood and *yang qi* concentrates around the stomach and intestine where it is needed for the digestive process. Any strong emotion or mental activity of any kind causes the *qi* and the blood to rise up to the head and so takes it away from the organs of digestion. This is why the habit of "working lunches" or grabbing a sandwich while doing business or even while driving the car is so bad for one's health. Not only is baby *yin* time being ignored but the digestive system is put under intense stress.

The importance of saliva has already been highlighted in the section on "Water as Medicine." Food should be thoroughly chewed and moistened with saliva before swallowing. Hot and cold food should not be mixed because the abrupt temperature changes will disturb the flow of blood and *qi* in the lining of the stomach. The teeth, too, often signal distress by becoming painfully sensitive to temperature changes.

You will remember that 11 A.M. to 1 P.M. is baby *yin* time. Eating properly and resting for at least half an hour after lunch ensures that baby *yin* is being well nourished. The quality of *qi* for the remainder of the day as well as the night's sleep to follow comes from the growth of baby *yin*.

When you first try taking a nap after lunch you may find yourself restless, with all the activities of the day still racing through your mind. Make sure you are warm, with a blanket over you if needed, and be patient with yourself. It often helps to do some gentle abdominal breathing. Alternatively, just accept that the mind will take a while, days or sometimes weeks, before it is convinced of this opportunity for rest. Before long, you will find yourself enjoying this half hour. When you lie down, a contented, dreamy feeling will come over you, and your whole body will feel deliciously warm and relaxed. If the routine is well established, you will find that even a short sleep of fifteen or twenty minutes leaves you alert and refreshed.

Many people get home after work in a state of exhaustion and pour themselves a glass of wine or spirits as a pick-me-up. The "heating" effect of the alcohol burns up more *yin qi*, resulting in a temporary excess of *yang* relative to *yin* that has the effect of stimulating the appetite (as in the western custom of aperitifs or cocktails). The result is often one of eating too much, too fast, and too late, all potent factors in obesity.

It is preferable to have a soft drink or a cup of tea when you come home after work, and then prepare something light and tasty to eat right away. Once the blood sugar recovers and the *qi* is flowing again, the desire for an alcoholic drink passes. The natural balance of *yin* and *yang* then regulates the appetite and there is no desire to overeat.

After the meal, make sure there is a further period of rest for at least half an hour. Sit quietly, or lie down. It helps to massage the tummy by moving the hand in a circular clockwise motion. Keep the mind calm and peaceful. Above all, don't watch violent or highly emotional television programs. Your sensitivity will increase as you improve your *qi*, and you will begin to notice that you instinctively avoid watching such programs. Ideally, a short, gentle walk to promote digestion should follow the period of rest. In contrast, exercise that is too vigorous after eating not only seriously depletes *yin qi* but also can cause chronic indigestion and irritable bowel syndrome.

The next consideration is what to eat. There are no rigid requirements in TCM because the whole approach is to listen to what your body is saying. If your body wants meat, then don't struggle to be a vegetarian. But remember, **information-*qi* is only accurate and reliable when your body-*qi* is strong and balanced.** If you are always craving chocolate, it does not follow that it is good to indulge in the habit. Any excessive desire points to an underlying imbalance of *qi* that first needs correcting. **If the *qi* is strong and balanced, cravings will simply disappear and so will the weight problem.**

If a variety of fresh foods is available, including fruits, vegetables, and cereals, the healthy body knows what it needs and will choose a mixture of foods that automatically provides the right balance of carbohydrates, fats, proteins, vitamins, and minerals. When the *qi* is strong, heavy or fatty foods are not appealing. The senses are sharpened and there is a desire for light, fresh food. This is why stir-fry vegetables are so appetizing. First wash the vegetables thoroughly, then chop them up and add to a preheated wok or saucepan containing a little very hot fat, preferably olive oil. Stir the vegetables for a couple of minutes until scorched on the outside, which sterilizes them. If they need further softening, just add a tablespoon or two of water and cover with a lid. The burst of steam cooks the vegetables throughout, and the little juice remaining is poured over the accompanying rice or noodles. Then nothing is wasted, the *qi* of the food is still strong, and all the vitamins are retained. (Boiling vegetables in water, or prolonged steaming, leaves you with food that has lost its natural color, lacks flavor, and has been drained of its nutrients.)

There are many books on stir-fry cuisine available. We will not deal with specific recipes here, but merely point out that what matters is the quality of the food. As the famous saying goes, we are what we eat!

Nature has arranged for the fruits and vegetables of the season to be the ones most beneficial for the corresponding time of the year. In hot weather, melons, cucumbers, tomatoes, and bananas are cooling. In colder weather, cabbage, pumpkin, and garlic are warming. While supermarkets these days offer almost all produce at any time, we need to remember that we are creatures of nature, designed over hundreds of thousands of years to follow the flow and rhythm of the seasons, and eating plenty of seasonal fruits and vegetables continues to be one of nature's best protections against illness.

These days, foods are defined above all by their energy content measured in calories (one calorie is the energy required to raise the temperature of one kilogram of water by one degree centigrade), and based on this measurement, each gram of fat yields nine calories and each gram of carbohydrate yields four. Consequently, many people think about food only in terms of calories. Yet experiments in Kirlian photography have demonstrated that the energy field of fresh food can be detected as a bioelectrical aura. Indeed, research using a combination of electrical sensors and ultrasound has demonstrated the presence of meridians in fruit, just as in the human body.

Freezing or overcooking food destroys the *qi* of the food. Precooked supermarket foods produce no Kirlian aura because the *qi* is long gone. On the other hand, the pure *qi* of fresh foods is absorbed directly into our bodies, the more so if our own *qi* is clean, since like attracts like. This is why Buddhist and Daoist monks, whose *qi* is very pure, can live for long periods on small quantities of nuts, fruits, or grain that would be way below subsistence levels if measured in calo-

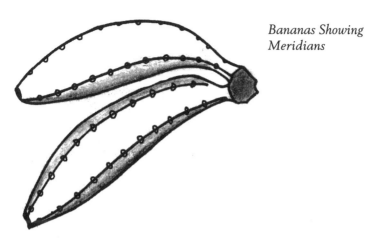

*Bananas Showing
Meridians*

ries. We can all benefit from a calm and peaceful mind that ensures that our body-*qi* is receptive to the *qi* of the food we eat. This is why it is so important to have relaxed, happy, and unhurried mealtimes.

In TCM, the art of nutrition is based on a balance of the five tastes, each one being associated with its internal organ as follows: sour/liver; bitter/heart; sweet/spleen; pungent/lung; and salty/kidney. These are linked in turn with specific cereals, fruits, animals, the five elements, and corresponding body parts according to the ancient Chinese tradition. Foods are also classified as "cooling," "neutral," and "warming" according to type. Together, this makes for a highly complex, interlocking system, for which the *Yellow Emperor's Canon of Medicine* remains the specialist's reference source. **Yet nothing could be simpler than the basic principle of aiming for a balance, which can be broadly achieved by using common sense, an awareness of the importance of variety, and the need to preserve *qi* in the preparation of food.** If you are suffering from an illness and are concerned with balancing your diet very accurately, it is best to consult a specialist in herbal TCM who will be able to diagnose your individual need. Once your *qi* is strong again, you can trust your body to be sensitive and let you know what it requires before you head for the store.

Natural Body Functions

ALL NATURAL BODY FUNCTIONS have a purpose. Just as a home needs chimneys and drains, so the body needs to keep its internal environment clean and healthy. When we need to belch or pass wind, it is because the air needs to be released. To hold back will only cause indigestion, chest pain, or cramps. If passing wind causes a smell, rather than feeling embarrassed it is better privately to congratulate your body on having successfully rid itself of toxins! The smell produced by this cleansing process soon passes, in any case. Another instance is when the stomach gurgles. People usually apologize and put a hand over the stomach to try to suppress the noise. In fact, gurgles are a good sign. They tell us that we need to eat, or that food is being digested as it should. Gurgles can also simply be a sign of relaxation.

Recently a journalist returned from a visit to China. He told how he had gone to the park early one morning and come across a beautiful young woman practicing "crane *qigong*." He had watched entranced, while oblivious of his presence she had performed her exercises with all the graceful and flowing movements of a bird in flight. Then the journalist confessed, "When she ended, what she did next really shocked me. She started belching and coughing and spitting on the ground, spoiling the whole effect!" The story shows how little the journalist had understood what he was seeing, for the young woman was quite properly cleansing herself of pathogenic *qi*, a sign that she had been doing good practice.

If you need to sneeze, don't hold back. Sneezing is the body's way of getting rid of pathogenic *qi*, by expelling germs from the nose and mouth, so sneezes should be allowed to come as nature intended. By all means, use a handkerchief to catch the germs but don't try to stifle the sneeze. Similarly, don't try to hide a yawn. Yawning is a sign that fresh *qi* needs taking in and stale *qi* needs expelling from the lungs. Check to see whether you need to do some abdominal breathing. Are you are genuinely tired, or is your body reacting to environment-*qi*? For instance, if you go to a meeting where people are busy mentally exhausting themselves, the deficiency of *qi* in the room may well start to drain your own *qi*. You may find that just being with someone who is very talkative but whose *qi* is low (as described under State Two in "Assessing the State of your Health") can induce a bout of yawning.

When you have a good yawn, either you will feel instantly refreshed (as cats do when they are rousing themselves) or else you will feel sleepier than ever, in which case close your eyes and doze for a little. Detach from your environment and enjoy a rest. If the problem is your own fatigue, you will concentrate all the better afterward. If it is because the environment-*qi* is low, you won't have missed much in any case. It is true that in the West you may have to contend with people feeling anxious or offended ("Am I boring you?") because the nature of *qi* is not understood. In China, yawning is more likely to be taken as a compliment since it is a sign that you feel free to relax.

If you need to pass urine, it is best to relieve yourself at the first opportunity. On the other hand, never try to force it either. The same applies to opening the bowels. Disturbing the natural rhythm of urination and defecation can affect the kidney meridian with several consequences: coldness of the knees and feet, hemorrhoids, lumbago, and, through the connection with the liver meridian, dryness of the eyes.

All these body functions are essential to life itself. Rather than feeling alienated from our bodies, we need to feel comfortable in them, valuing and respecting the complex processes on which our daily health depends.

Medicinal Plants

SOME MEDICINAL PLANTS have a place in traditional western medicine. The common foxglove, or *Digitalis*, for example, contains an active constituent widely prescribed for the treatment of certain heart conditions. In China almost all foods, plants, and herbs have a place in the medical pharmacopoeia, with more than five thousand preparations. Over as many thousand years, there have been detailed studies of their medicinal properties, their effect on *qi* and the meridians, and their beneficial and toxic properties. For minor ailments, certain plants can be used singly. On most occasions, accurate mixing of a number of plants is required depending on the clinical condition of the individual patient. There are over sixty-one thousand combinations of plants to choose from. Not surprisingly, specialization in botanical Chinese medicine requires deep knowledge and years of intensive study.

It is unwise to make blanket recommendations about plant remedies. Ginseng, for instance, can be a very effective treatment for certain conditions, especially when *yang qi* is very weak due to illness or old age. But in the wrong circumstances, such as in the cases of *yin* deficiency so common in the West, taking ginseng as a casual remedy can cause palpitations, nervousness, restlessness, and even bleeding from the nose. A specialist should prescribe the treatment of specific disorders with botanical medicines only after examination and diagnosis. Preventative medicine is part of daily life in China, where families routinely prepare botanical mixtures for daily consumption to promote health and longevity. An old Chinese story tells of the virtues of one such preparation, *xunlaowan*.

In ancient China, an official happened to be riding through a village close by Zhongnan Mountain when he saw a woman in her thirties upbraiding a man who looked about one hundred years old and giving him a sound beating with a stick. The official dismounted and inquired what was going on. When he was told that the old man was the woman's son, he was astonished. He had the woman summoned and asked her what she was up to.

She replied, "In our family we have had a magic prescription handed down from generation to generation that is taken to prevent aging. I was rebuking my son because try as I might, he would never listen to me and take the prescription as he was told. That is why his back is bent and his hair has grown white. I'm very angry about it!" After hearing this, the official begged for the prescription for himself. He took it regularly and just as expected, his physical strength increased, his silver hair turned black once more, his face became smooth like a child's, and he lived to a great age!

Xunlaowan is difficult to obtain because some of its ingredients are rare, even in China, and the preparation is complex. *Heshouwu*, which is the tuber of the Chinese fleece flower (*Polygonatum multiflorum*) and one of the key plants in *xunlaowan*, nourishes both *yin* and *yang* and is used to retain youthfulness, reduce cholesterol levels, strengthen heart function, and promote healthy bowel movements. *Heshouwu* can be obtained in the West from Chinese medical and herbal shops. In China, it is taken in "immortal porridge," made by boiling thirty to sixty grams of *heshouwu* in water with sixty grams of rice, three to five large red Chinese dates, and sugar to taste. This recipe is used for deficiency of *yang* in the liver and kidney and also for anemia.

There are two other important botanical ingredients in *xunlaowan*—*dihuang* (*Rehmannia glutinosa*) and *gouqizi*, or Chinese wolfberry (*Lycium chinense*), both of which are good for the treatment of *yin* deficiency. These can be readily obtained from Chinese medical and herbal shops. *Dihuang* can be bought prepacked as *liuwei dihuang wan*. It comes as a black substance the size of a large marble, contained in a wax shell that must to be squeezed hard to crack open. A TCM examination is needed before taking this medication, because the dose and duration of the treatment will depend on the nature and severity of the *yin* deficiency. *Dihuang* strengthens the heart, liver, and kidneys, nourishes the *yin* and the blood, and is used for the treatment of tinnitus, dizziness, palpitations, insomnia, backache, hot flushes, and night sweats.

Gouqizi can be purchased loose as small, red, dried berries that have a pleasant taste and can be sprinkled on porridge. Alternatively, it comes prepacked in wax balls as *qijiu dihuang*, again best taken on specific TCM advice. *Gouqizi* strengthens liver and kidneys and is used to treat dizziness, headache, and blurred vision.

Certain plants can be used very simply to restore the balance of heat and cold according to the weather. For instance, if you go out and get caught in wind and rain, on your return take off the wet clothes immediately, dry the body, and have some warm ginger tea. This is made by combining thinly sliced root ginger (about nine grams) and brown sugar (twelve grams) in a pan with a cupful of gently boiling water for a few minutes; add one or two sliced spring onions just before pouring. As soon as you drink this, you will feel your stomach glowing, and this feeling will spread to the whole body. You will then begin to sweat lightly and perhaps sneeze a few times. Taken right away, this drink will prevent the onset of a cold since the "heat" in the ingredients will drive out any pathogenic *qi* that may have entered.

Ginger is widely used in China. It promotes the circulation of blood and warms the whole body, activates the meridians, nourishes the five internal organs, and strengthens the lower *dantian*. It can treat stomachache and detoxify the aftereffects of alcohol. In China it is used in cooking seafood and meat because it also protects against food poisoning. Ginger should be avoided in hot weather, as should any strongly pungent herbal or plant remedy.

During the summer, heat causes such problems as excessive sweating, thirst, dryness of the eyes, and headache. Chrysanthemum tea, made by pouring boiling water over a pinch or two of the dried flowers, is particularly cooling. It is also used in the treatment of coronary heart disease and high blood pressure because these conditions are characterized by excess "heat."

Autumn is a time when the weather is cooling but the body may still be carrying the heat of the summer. According to TCM, internal heat can cause inflammation of the respiratory tract, and people who have weak lung *qi* are at risk of getting asthma, colds, and skin disorders (the latter because of the connection of the lung meridian with the skin). The whole body needs to be gently cooled in step with the change of season, and pears are the best fruit for this purpose. They penetrate the lung meridian, cleaning the lungs, dispersing any excess heat, and relieving any cough or dryness of the throat.

Spring onion and red date tea is a pleasant drink that strengthens the heart and calms the mind. First wash and soak about twenty Chinese red dates until they swell; then vigorously boil them for twenty minutes in a pan of water. Add the white bulbs of about seven spring onions with roots still attached and simmer for ten minutes more. Drink one cup of this tea in the morning and one cup in the evening. The white part of the spring onion is warming in nature and goes to the lungs and stomach. *Yang qi* is strengthened, internal stagnation is relieved, and migraines, abdominal pain, and constipation are alleviated. Red dates are sweet and strengthen spleen *qi*, nourish the blood (good for anemia), improve the skin, calm the mind, and relieve insomnia. Because they promote the flow of *qi*, they can also relieve pain due to blockages of *qi*.

Drinking Alcohol:
Vice or Virtue?

NO DRINK HAS ATTRACTED more praise and greater condemnation than alcohol. Mankind has used alcohol since the ancient discovery of the natural fermentation of sugars by yeast. Alcohol has been used in China medically as well as socially for over four thousand years. Consequently, its effects for good and ill have been closely investigated, with the result that from the TCM perspective there are very clear rules about the right way and the wrong way to drink.

Li Shizhen, a famous physician during the Ming dynasty, pronounced, "Wine is indeed a delicious drink bestowed by Heaven. Drinking it properly helps the blood and *qi* circulate, invigorates the mind, eases mental stress, and adds to the pleasure of life. Drinking without restraint impairs the mind, the blood, and the stomach *qi*, producing internal heat which leads at best to disease and at worst to the humiliation of the nation, the ruin of the family, and the loss of life!"

The Chinese term "wine" means not only the fermented grape but also fermented cereals (rice wine, for example) and all spirits. As a nutrient, wine is classed as warm in nature, pungent, and both bitter and sweet in taste. In excess, alcohol is a poison, but used with care it is strongly medicinal, vitalizing the spleen, liver, stomach, and small intestine, expelling pathogenic wind and cold, and promoting circulation of the blood and *qi*. Being pure *yang*, it penetrates quickly to all regions of the body including the skin and is therapeutic for rheumatic conditions and other painful disorders, including post trauma. The Chinese also use spirits such as whiskey as a solvent for other medicinal ingredients—the herb *gouqizi*, for example, which is used for strengthening the liver and kidney. This is known as medicated wine and can be taken regularly in small quantities after meals.

Recent medical research has shown that a small amount of wine taken daily (one to two glasses) can have a protective effect on the heart and circulatory system, confirming the advice of the sages of ancient China. Similarly, it is now well known that too much alcohol damages the stomach and liver. TCM emphasizes that the resulting "excess heat" harms the very organs that benefit from a smaller, therapeutic dose.

A cardinal rule in TCM is that wine should never be drunk on an empty stomach. The alcohol is instantly absorbed through the lining of the stomach into the blood stream, and being pure *yang*, it disperses rapidly throughout the body and opens the pores of the skin. *Yin qi* is burned up by the powerful internal heating effect, as well as leaking out through the skin. As a result, the body rapidly becomes *yin* deficient.

Someone who is *yin* deficient is likely to feel irritable and restless, craving stimulation to ward off underlying tiredness. This is how a vicious circle arises, with the temptation to use alcohol as a pick-me-up. Sleep is affected, with the insomnia, disturbed dreams, and night sweats characteristic of *yin* deficiency, so that baby *yang* cannot be nourished and the next day starts depleted of *yang*. This is how reliance on alcohol at lunchtime to boost *yang* often begins, leading to the whole cycle of alcohol abuse.

Thirst should always be quenched with fresh water, tea, or natural fruit juice, for not only is fluid being replaced but also the body itself benefits from the "cool" character of the beverage.

The correct way to drink wine is during or after a meal, making sure that there is already some food in the stomach. All too often, people drink for an immediate lift. A different process takes place when good quality wine is sipped unhurriedly during a relaxed meal. Digestion is encouraged, the circulation of the blood and *qi* is improved, and the internal organs are vitalized. The quality of the wine is crucial, for the better the wine, the better will be its *qi*. Cheap wines, especially those with chemical additives, are to be avoided. Spirits over ten years old will guarantee a fine, pure *qi* that is especially beneficial.

Getting drunk is dangerous, for as well as causing *yin* and *yang* deficiency, at this level the alcohol is acting as a neurotoxin. For over two thousand years it has been customary in China for a host to offer strong green tea to a guest who has drunk too much. Green tea works by cleansing the body of accumulated excess heat. Several cups will usually overcome the symptoms of intoxication within an hour and protect against any hangover.

Q*i* and Sex

$\mathcal{S}$EX BETWEEN a woman and a man offers a life-giving exchange of *yin* and *yang*, resulting in a strong *qi*, resistance to illness, and an increased longevity. These benefits occur when the right conditions are fulfilled. If sex is used carelessly, or in excess, we are warned that far from improving health, we will be risking illness and a shortening of life expectancy.

For more than two thousand years, Daoists have held that sex should take place within a stable and loving relationship. In 1978, research was carried out in China in the district of Bamaxian, famous for its long-lived inhabitants. The survey demonstrated that everyone who remained fit and well over the age of ninety had enjoyed harmonious and loving marriages.

The TCM view is that a couple should not engage in sex until both have reached adulthood. This is because mature males and females produce sexual secretions that are rich in *jing*, a precious essence made from kidney *qi*. The purpose of the sexual act, besides conception, is for each partner to attain a merging of *yin* and *yang* with the *jing*. The man receives from the woman the *yin qi* of her vaginal juices and gives in return the *yang qi* of his prostatic juices and sperm. In this way, each attains the correct balance of *yin* and *yang*, ensuring long-lasting vigor and freedom from disease. Optimally, the man's sperm must be mature and copious, while for the woman, the best time for sex is from the second day after her menstrual period ends, allowing time for her to recover her *yin* after the blood loss.

This exchange of *qi* does not require ejaculation; indeed, for the most part it is best avoided. Consequently, the sexual act can be experienced and enjoyed in a very different way from simply making orgasm the aim and measure of success. Sun Simiao, a great physician and *qigong* master who lived during the Tung dynasty in the seventh century, gave this advice:

Before lovemaking, breathing should be relaxed; the man and woman should be filled with happiness and through kissing and embracing become attuned to each other. As the *qi* rises, more saliva flows and in kissing, they exchange and swallow each other's saliva. [Saliva is regarded as a precious juice; see "Water as Medicine."] The *qi* continues to rise as shown in the woman by reddening of the face (heart *qi*), bodily movements (spleen *qi*), warming of the nose (lung *qi*), shining eyes (liver *qi*) and moistening of the vagina (kidney *qi*). In the man, the rising *qi* is shown by the first stirrings of the penis (liver *qi*), enlargement and heat of the penis (heart *qi*) and finally stiffness (kidney *qi*).

Only then must the penis be introduced, slowly and without force. Calm breathing should be maintained, assisted by breathing in through the nose and slowly out through the mouth. There should be no sudden, thrusting movement that might disturb the *qi* of the five internal organs. Exertion and sweating should be avoided to preserve *qi*. As the penis deeply enters the woman, the couple should both focus on the lower dantian, visualizing it as a glowing red ball about the size of a hen's egg. This will intensify the *qi* and reduce the desire for orgasm. If the man feels close to ejaculation, he should withdraw, no matter how often, be it ten times or more and as part of love making, the sensation of reintroducing the penis will give both partners cause for renewed pleasure.

When the man lies still, deep inside the woman, they are embracing both externally and internally. The kidney *qi* responds by rising to the face and the couple should then lie mouth-to-mouth, exchanging saliva and gently moving together. The eyes should be closed, the breathing quiet and the body relaxed. *Qi* is now flowing between the couple; the man is drinking the *yin* and the woman the *yang*. This is a time of great intimacy, which is also one of sharing together in the *yin* and *yang* of the cosmos. When it feels right to conclude the act of sex, the couple lie together peacefully, feeling vitalized with strong *qi*.

A second way recommended by the ancient texts for a couple to merge their *yin* and *yang* does not even require genital contact. The couple lie together embracing and holding hands and visualize drawing in clean, fresh *qi* with each breath. Then they concentrate on the *qi* as it moves from the hands to the elbows, armpits, shoulder, neck, and face, down the chest to the lower *dantian* and from there up the spine to the head. All the while, the couple gaze into each other's eyes, linking them very powerfully in spirit *(shen qi)*. This leads to a profound experience, for the sense of personal self yields to a merging with the whole cosmos.

Apart from these specific techniques, just the simple act of spending the night together in a loving embrace will enable a couple to exchange *yin* and *yang* while they sleep.

There are clear guidelines in TCM about the ejaculation of sperm. In general, not more than twice a month is advised because of the loss of *qi*. Other considerations include the man's health and age. The ancient texts give the following advice: for a man of twenty years, once in four days; at thirty, once in eight days; at forty, once in sixteen days; at fifty, once in twenty days; and at sixty, if the *qi* is strong, once a month.

In addition, both the man and woman can use their information-*qi* to see whether the loss of *qi* is within safe limits. If after sex the body feels comfortable and rested, the mind relaxed and happy, and the brain alert and efficient, the body-*qi* is still strong. If the back feels sore and there is the sensation of physical or mental fatigue, it means the *qi* has been drained. Sometimes, despite this, there is a feeling of restlessness and the urge to engage in sex again. If so, remember the telltale signs of State Two in "Assessing the State of your Health," when the *qi* is "noisy" but half empty. The *yin*-deficient person is quick to get aroused and the sex drive may appear to be strong but the energy soon flags. More generally, sex leading to orgasm when either person is fatigued is detrimental to health.

The symptoms of exhaustion of *qi* due to sex follow the same

broad pattern as shown in the graph of information-*qi* (see page 40)
and include dizziness, visual problems, breathlessness, backache,
abdominal pain and inflammation, cessation of periods in the
woman, and impotence in the man. In western society, the most
common danger arises from starting sex too young and keeping it
going excessively (sometimes obsessively) throughout adulthood
while remaining *qi* deficient throughout. The consequence is premature aging, sexual burnout by midlife, vulnerability to disease,
and a shortening of the life span.

**Sex in accordance with Daoist teachings, on the other hand, can
only be beneficial. If there is restraint concerning orgasm, the *qi*
will continue to flow with all the vigor of youth. The desire to
make love continues unabated for the whole of the lifetime,
bestowing on the couple all the benefits of health, intimacy,
happiness, and perpetual youthfulness.**

As with all matters of body-*qi*, the environment-*qi* needs to be
taken into account. Sex should be avoided in stormy weather because of pathogenic *qi*, as well as when it is excessively hot or cold,
in direct sunlight or moonlight, and in places where it would be
wrong to make love, such as churches or graveyards. All these situations will influence the subtle exchange of *yin* and *yang* between
the couple. Other factors to bear in mind are that the couple
should neither be hungry, when *qi* will be low, nor overfull because
of the concentration of *qi* and blood in the stomach. If the emotions are running high, whether anger, fear or overelation, or there
is excessive worry for any reason, the flow of *qi* will be affected.
Sex should never be forced because it can never result in a harmonious blending of *yin* and *yang*.

Sex and alcohol together are to be avoided, from the TCM perspective. Sex uses up *yang qi* in three ways, internally because of the
physical exertion, externally by leaking from the surface of the body
due to the opening of the pores of the skin and, last but not least,
through the loss of sexual secretions. Alcohol, being pure *yang*, increases both the internal heat and the transport of *qi* to the surface

of the body. The mental and physical excitement that results is short-lived and followed by a lowering of *qi*, opening the door to pathogenic *qi* and to the syndrome of *qi* deficiency as described under State Two in "Assessing the State of Your Health." In this condition, the overarousal, which masks underlying *qi* deficiency, may stimulate further sexual activity, another vicious circle in which kidney *qi* is drained. At the very least, this leads to back problems. (The saying "the best form of exercise for the lower back is sex" is far from true.) More seriously, the meridians are damaged, the immune system is weakened and life-threatening diseases can take hold.

What holds for alcohol goes for any other mood-enhancing drug. The rising *qi* that leads naturally to sex comes from a state of deep relaxation, which is possible only when the *qi* is full. The use of drugs may enable two people to engage in the mechanics of sex, but their *qi* will be deeply disturbed and their health is certain to suffer.

According to TCM, there should be no sex during the menstrual period because the woman's *qi* will already be drained. Nor should it be attempted when either person has been suffering from an acute illness. When the woman is pregnant, she should conserve her *qi* for the baby during the first and last three months of the pregnancy and abstain from sex for one hundred days after childbirth (while her *yin* is recovering from the blood loss). Breast-feeding also requires the *qi* and the blood for milk production.

When a couple wants to conceive, by respecting and valuing the principles of TCM, they will be making a nourishing and happy home for the new member of the family from the very start. Their strong and balanced *qi* ensures that the sperm will swim vigorously, the egg will be ready, and the womb will be welcoming. The mother's lower *dantian* will bathe the baby in its full, warm *qi* throughout the pregnancy, and when the time comes, the baby will be born into its new life with all the advantages nature can provide.

The Daoist teachings make clear that most people will experience their sex drive as a normal part of life that needs to be accommodated like any other natural instinct. The art is in knowing how to promote health and happiness in doing so. Imposing abstinence only leads to trouble since frustration and resentment are potent causes of damage to the *qi*. Throughout history, there has always been a minority of people who are indifferent to sex because their energy is given instead to a spiritual discipline. In the case of certain *qigong* masters working at the highest level, the fusion of their own internal *yin* and *yang* supersedes the need to merge *qi* through making love. Instead, the body merges with the *taiji* of the cosmos.

Traveling with Ease

ALL OUR LIVES we are immersed in environment-*qi*, and any major disturbance of it is bound to affect us. This needs to be taken into account when we travel. Storms, high winds, lightning, heavy rain, or fog all occur when the balance of the *yin* and *yang* of the climate is temporarily disturbed. Because of modern technology, we take less notice of these fluctuations in environment-*qi* than did our forebears. Sitting warm and dry in a car or plane insulates us from the power of the elements, and we may feel secure in our comfort. At the same time, we know from news reports that major accidents often occur in storm conditions, when the natural world demonstrates its raw power by tossing around cars, planes, and ships as though they were mere toys.

Further, our own *qi* can be directly disturbed by the state of the environment-*qi*. Everyone knows that it is dangerous to go out during a thunderstorm, but in spite of this, people still go out of doors during storms, sometimes with the disastrous consequence of being struck by lightning. Far from protecting themselves, they have become caught up in the power of the *qi* and expose themselves to its danger as if under a spell. Another example is what the police call "motorway madness," when drivers seem to defy all common sense by driving at high speeds in fog or rain, resulting in multiple pileups.

If possible, postpone your journey until the weather has improved. The more upset the environment-*qi*, the greater the need to remain calm. It is best to sit quietly at home, closing the doors and windows to ensure that your own *qi* is balanced and harmonious.

Maintaining this inner calmness not only helps you to stay detached from imbalances in environment-*qi* but directly helps protect you when you run into unforeseen situations that put you at risk. The following advice comes from Sun Simiao: "If you plan to travel to wild parts, before you set off, chant the mantra *jin sha jia lou*. You will lessen the chance of falling into danger. If you should encounter thieves or bandits, at once calm yourself and strengthen your *qi* by chanting the mantra a further two times. You will lessen the chance of becoming a victim." This mantra (for which there is no translation) was first used by the disciples of the Buddha twenty-five hundred years ago. It is understood to work by enabling the person to create a special *qi*, so strong that it radiates to the source of danger and overcomes the threat.

In the industrialized world, the dangers of travel are more likely to be caused by exhaustion from crowded and stressful conditions that lower the *qi* and pave the way for infections and illnesses. Another important factor is air pollution, including significant reduction in the oxygen level in crowded trains and pressurized airplanes.

The best way to cope with this situation is to reduce your own oxygen needs. Remember that mental activity adds to your oxygen need, so switch off your mobile phone and your laptop computer and calm your mind. Whether you are standing or sitting, close your eyes and begin practicing abdominal breathing, nourishing your *qi*, and slowing down your own metabolic demands. If it helps to have music, put on your Walkman and listen to music that is gentle and soothing. You are now taking the opportunity of turning a high-stress event into a stress-relieving occasion.

The same principle applies to flights, especially long ones where there is likely to be jet lag. If you start watching in-flight videos or reading exciting novels, you will not relax and doze off. Instead, you will be affected by the commotion of travel and the presence of other people in a confined space. The physiological arousal will heighten your appetite so that you will be likely to eat and drink more. Drinking alcohol will risk increasing your internal heat and your loss of *qi* at a time when you most need to conserve them. Similarly, because of the reduced oxygen level in the aircraft, the body must work harder to digest food. The end result is that you leave the aircraft a good deal more tired than when you embarked.

The disruption to your biorhythms is minimized the closer you can come to a state of hibernation. For the duration of the journey, leave flying the plane to the pilot and allow yourself to be carried like a baby! Close your eyes, relax, and doze. You will feel less hungry and thirsty, and you will give your body the chance to make its own adaptation to the changing time zones while you rest. If at some point you do decide to read, make sure it is something light. (Newspapers are generally full of gloom and doom.)

If you must drive to your destination, leave plenty of time for the journey so that you are not continually frustrated by the traffic. Build in a break so that you can get out of the car and stretch your legs or have some light refreshment. If you feel sleepy, recline the seat and have a doze. Because you are taking the pressure off yourself, you will become more sensitive to your information-*qi*. Allow yourself to be guided by your own *qi* rather than external demands. If a traffic jam or an accident spoils your plans to get somewhere by a certain time, the key lies in acceptance. Since there is nothing you can do to change it, you may as well relax.

When you reach your destination, have a warm shower at the first opportunity. Apart from washing off the grime of the journey, it will restore the circulation and the flow of *qi* in the meridians that may well have stagnated. If there is no shower, sit and relax with your feet in a bowl of warm water. This will directly stimulate the six major meridians that begin or end in the feet, activate kidney *qi*, and nourish the internal organs.

Last, physical sprains and bruises are not uncommon while traveling. Often a pack of ice is applied in the belief that it will hasten recovery. However, the TCM approach is to regard the redness, heat, and swelling as part and parcel of nature's healing response. The blood flow increases so that cells involved in the repair work can be transported to the site of injury and the dead cells removed.

Along with the blood, the *qi* is mobilized to promote rapid recovery. Chilling or freezing will only slow this process down. The solution is to stay calm and rest the injured part so that nature can get on with the job of healing. If there happens to be a TCM doctor available, acupressure or acupuncture will speed the recovery.

Keeping Your Home
from Harm

JUST AS YOUR MIND dwells within the body, so your body
dwells in your home. It therefore follows you should treat your
home with the same care and respect that you give your body
and apply the same principles of good sense and moderation. Your
home should be pleasantly warm and dry. If the weather is fine, windows should be left open so that fresh air can circulate freely. When
the weather is poor, at least open the windows for a short while
morning and evening (and lunchtime if you are staying in during the
day). Dampness and draughts render the body vulnerable to pathogenic *qi*, which can cause various illnesses, from infections and colds
to facial paralysis and strokes. Even the most beautiful house cannot
offer your body the protection it needs if it stands in a location suffering from heavy pollution.

According to the ancient text of the *Yijing*, the ideal house faces
south, nestling on the lower slopes of the south face of a mountain.
The house catches the sunlight all year round and being slightly ele-
vated, it makes the most of winter sunlight when the arc of the sun
is lower in the sky. Beyond the garden in the front of the house flows
a river, winding around the foot of the mountain. The effect of the
water is to stabilize and maintain environment-*qi* (similar to the way
a capacitor stores electricity) while the house is protected from the

chill of the north wind. (The name of the ancient skill of *fengshui* means wind / water in Chinese.)

Few of us have the good fortune to be able to live in such a place. But there are some basic considerations to keep in mind when choosing where to live. From the TCM perspective it helps to find somewhere with a garden, or a park close to hand, with trees, vegetation, and a peaceful atmosphere. This is more important than putting style first. The location should be sheltered, with good access to sunlight and with light airy rooms. We also need to trust our intuition as to whether the *qi* in a house "feels right," something which we often sense the moment we step through the door.

Inside, the house should be furnished simply. The ancient texts warn us that having too many ornate and expensive possessions will simply invite robbery. Nor should the house be too big for its occupants, for there needs to be a balance between the space it provides and the number of people within. Elderly people remaining alone in a large house, which once rang with the noise and laughter of a family, are putting themselves at risk of pathogenic *qi* because they are not producing enough of the *yang* "doing" to balance the *yin* "being" of the house. It is better to live in a house where there is a comfortable fit, just as we take care to choose the right size of shoe for the foot.

The sage Sun Simiao, whose advice we gave concerning traveling to remote places, also recommends a specific procedure when moving to a new home that ensures that the *qi* of the house is strengthened and will provide protection against burglary. "When you rise on the second day, clean your mouth with fresh water. Then burn incense all round the house. In each room first stand in the southeast corner, facing southwest, and then chant '*jin sha jia lou*' while walking to the southwest corner. Walk back chanting '*ni zi shuo yang*' and do this seven times."

Houses absorb the *qi* of the inhabitants, so it is important to start with a clean slate and safeguard the *qi* of your home by maintaining an atmosphere of relaxation and calm. Not only will you benefit, but the security and safety of your house will also be enhanced even when you have to be away from home.

Preparing for Sleep

ANIMALS VARY IN THE AMOUNT of sleep they need, from none, as with dolphins, to cats that spend more time asleep than awake. Humans spend up to one third of their lives sleeping, but there is a good deal of individual variation. Some people thrive on only four or five hours a night while others need eight hours or more. What really matters is the quality. Waking from sleep, whether it be four or eight hours, and finding yourself still tired and listless means that the sleep has been shallow and the body has not been replenished.

There has been extensive research on brain activity during sleep. For the first ninety minutes, sleep deepens steadily until we are in what is called stage four sleep, characterized by slow brain waves and during which we are difficult to rouse. Then after a further ninety minutes we enter REM (rapid eye movements) sleep, during which the brain waves become faster, the heart rate increases, and there is often visible twitching of muscles. REM sleep is associated with vivid dreaming. It accounts for about one quarter of sleep time, alternating with slow-wave sleep. As the night goes on, slow-wave sleep gives way to increasing REM sleep, and it is from REM sleep that we usually wake.

It is evident that sleep is a time of highly organized brain activity vital to our health. Research has shown that during slow-wave sleep, growth hormone is released from the pituitary gland beneath the brain, stimulating not only growth but also fat and protein

151

metabolism essential to the repair and renewal of body tissues. REM sleep is thought to exercise the whole neural network, necessary for the maintenance of the circuitry of the central nervous system. Also during sleep the pineal body, an outgrowth of the brain, synthesizes the hormone melatonin, needed for the functioning of the thyroid, adrenal, and sex reproductive glands.

Caffeine, alcohol, and many other drugs disturb the internal rhythm of the sleeping brain. Lack of REM sleep causes loss of concentration, memory, and learning capacity. Total sleep deprivation rapidly unbalances the mind, and if continued for more than two weeks it will result in total physical collapse and even death.

If we have properly prepared for sleep, we drift off peacefully within a few minutes of going to bed. Sleeping during baby *yang* time, between 11 P.M. and 1 A.M. coincides with the first period of slow-wave sleep, when essential body repairs are taking place. When we awake refreshed, energetic, clear-headed, and ready for the day ahead, we know that the body has been fully able to carry out its maintenance program overnight.

On the other hand, if we long for sleep but night after night find ourselves tossing and turning, or waking during the night with disturbing dreams and in a sweat, or lying awake during the small hours feeling exhausted but unable to relax, we need to face the fact that not only is this highly distressing, it also means that we are seriously injuring our health.

Preparing for sleep brings together a number of key points common to the principles of TCM health care. Each day needs to be lived with an awareness of the *taiji*. Baby *yin* needs nourishing with a rest or sleep at lunchtime so that *yin qi* can grow throughout the afternoon and evening. This means avoiding strenuous exercise in the evening, especially during kidney meridian time (5 to 7 P.M.), as well as excessive mental arousal including emotional excitement, television programs or films that are overstimulating, and caffeine or alcohol. Any worrying should be postponed to the next day when *yang* can be employed to help resolve the problem. The evening meal should be unhurried and enjoyed, not too large and not too late in the day. A bath or a shower is normally not needed every day but when taken, it should be in good time to allow for relaxation afterward. Washing must always include bathing the buttocks and feet in warm water. It is important after washing to wear socks or slippers so the feet stay warm until bedtime; neither should the body be allowed to get cold. If there is a sleep problem, now is the time to spend half an hour relaxing. Calm the mind by doing some meditation or gentle *qigong* movements if you know them. (There is an ancient saying, "First put your mind to sleep and the body will follow.") Be in bed by 11 P.M. at the latest. All these preparations will ensure that *yin* has grown undisturbed and full and will enable your sleep to be deep and restful.

The bedroom should be clean, with fresh air, and neither too warm or too cool. Between 60 and 68 degrees Fahrenheit (16 to 20 degrees centigrade) is suitable. The air should not be too dry, so that the nose and throat are protected from drying up during the night. The bed should be level and the mattress firm. The blankets or duvet should be light but sufficiently warm to maintain body temperature without sweating. When the *qi* is strong, there is no need for a hot-water bottle. If one is used, it should not be too hot and should rest against the feet.

The head should be uncovered and away from any draught, window, radiator, or fire. As to the direction of the bed, there are two options to try. The first is to have the head toward the east during the *yang* seasons of spring and summer in order to benefit from the *yang qi* of the rising sun, and to the west for the *yin* seasons of autumn and winter so that the head is nourished by the *yin*. The second method is always to have the head toward the east. (Avoid lying with the head toward the north, which in TCM is associated with health problems due to excess *yin*).

When in bed, keep the mouth closed. Sleeping with an open mouth causes loss of *qi*, as well as drying out the mouth, nose, and throat, and encouraging snoring. (When the *qi* is weak, the jaw tends to drop open at night.) It is best to start the night by lying on the right side, which alleviates pressure on the heart. Have the knees gently bent. This opens the liver meridians as they pass up the inside of the leg and improves liver functioning during the night. (The liver acts as a reservoir for pooled blood, promotes digestion, and acts on the *qi*, preventing stagnation and maintaining a smooth flow throughout the body.)

During pregnancy, it is advisable to lie on the left side because the majority of wombs are positioned asymmetrically, and lying on the left side relieves pressure on the right ureter and major blood vessels.

Deep and restful sleep is characterized by rapid onset, slow rhythmic breathing without snoring, absence of disturbing dreams, sleeping right through to the morning, and waking with a clear mind and a body ready and willing to begin the day. Following the principles of *Listen to Your Body* will ensure you get a good night's sleep.

Enjoy Aging with
the Help of Your *Qi*

IN **ЛHITOU ЛHAN**, a remote village in the Liaoning province of China, lives a man called Li Xiangyang. Li is often out and about on his bicycle. He is sound of wind and limb and walks with a straight back and a firm step. His eyes are keen, his hearing acute, his voice strong, and his mind clear. He worked for most of his life as a laborer and builder. Now retired, he continues to exercise, going for walks three times a day throughout spring, summer, and autumn. Li's home, which he keeps clean and tidy, is simple in character but sufficient for his needs. He maintains a lifelong habit of three regular meals a day with plenty of rice porridge and fresh vegetables, always finishing the meal "just 80 percent full." Then he massages his tummy and makes sure to stretch his limbs.

It is cold in the winter in the north of China. Li stays home, equally content to be on his own or have members of his family visit. This can keep him busy at times since he has, at the last count, ninety-nine living descendants. Li's son is 78, his grandson 57, great-grandson 29, and great-great grandson 9 years old.

Li is 102 years old. When asked how he has managed to stay so fit and well, he says it is quite simple. "My mind is calm and I live my life without regrets. I never made a profit at someone else's expense and so I have nothing to reproach myself for." He won't be drawn into anger. "That's why my heart has never been diseased."

What gives him pleasure? "Helping others—it makes life meaningful and interesting." What about times when he is alone? He replies, "I am so happy to have no worries that I often just laugh aloud even by myself!" Here is great wisdom coming from a simple man.

Li shares much in common with many other centenarians in China who have been the subject of considerable research. In Jilin province lives Fu Cai, who is 125 years old. He recently received an award for his achievements as a "model worker in forestry for over one hundred years"!

One study looked at 865 centenarians in Xinjiang province and 54 in Zhejiang province. The subjects exhibited the following defining characteristics:

- They share a lifetime habit of light to moderate physical work. Many of the centenarians came from the countryside and worked in the fields. They continue with their physical activities, which include walking, jogging, and doing fitness exercises or *qigong*.

- They are honest, broadminded, optimistic, and happy by nature. They remain emotionally calm and peaceful, showing no signs of anxiety or frustration. They are not competitive or materialistic but content with the basic necessities of life.

- They value a simple and regular routine in their daily lives.

- There were almost no smokers in the study. A minority sip a small glass of wine with the evening meal.

- The great majority are vegetarian, make a point of eating in moderation, and drink several cups of green tea daily.

- They engage in recreational pursuits that maintain their mental activity and involvement in life: chess, calligraphy and painting, writing, music, gardening, and fishing.

This research bears out the wisdom of a hundred generations. Calm mind and healthy body work together as one. Day-by-day quality, based on the principles of TCM, leads to year-after-year good health. Young people in the modern world rarely have either the knowledge or the foresight to live according to these principles. Only later, when a health problem occurs, does the picture change, bringing with it the realization that life can no longer be taken for granted and that the body is mortal.

This painful awareness can be the start of a rebirth. If we have the necessary information on which to act and the will to do so, we can learn how to listen to the body and how to look after its needs. We will be rewarded handsomely.

Postscript

Fame or self: Which matters more?
Self or wealth: Which is more precious?
Gain or loss: Which is more painful?

He who is attached to things will suffer much.
He who saves will suffer heavy loss.
A contented man is never disappointed.
He who knows when to stop does not find himself in trouble.
He will stay forever safe.

      —Laozi, *Daodejing*

NOW THAT YOU HAVE READ this book, pause and reflect on what you have learned. Can you recognize yourself in these pages? If so, what changes do you need to make to your life?

This book has been written so that you can know, even before visible illness has occurred, how to be well and stay well. The inspiration for the book came from patients who, on recovering their health, suggested that such a book could make a big difference to the lives of friends and family. Many have said that if only they had known about these things before, no end of suffering could have been avoided.

Everyone deserves the chance to benefit from the wisdom and advice to be found in these pages. The title *Listen to Your Body* was

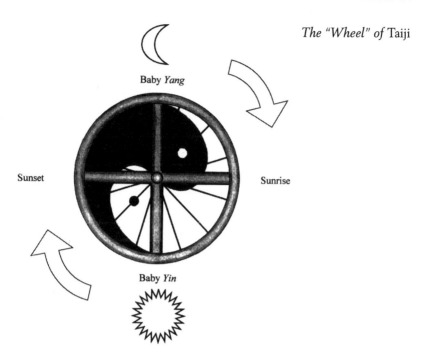

The "Wheel" of Taiji

chosen because that wisdom is already within you. You are the doctor and this book is here to assist you.

You may be asking, "There is so much to do, where and how should I begin?" Start by thinking of your life as a wheel that turns on four main spokes. First be sure to nourish baby *yang* by preparing for bedtime with a calm mind and body. Have a shower or bath, or at least a footbath, followed by some time to do abdominal breathing and be in bed by 11.00 P.M. (gall bladder meridian time 11.00 P.M.– 1.00 A.M.). By nurturing your baby *yang,* you will wake at sunrise, energetic and alert.

Now you have the opportunity, between 5 A.M. and 9 A.M. (large intestine and stomach meridian times) to do your *qigong* practice and any other physical exercise you may like, out of doors if possible. Remember to enjoy a good breakfast without hurrying. *Yang qi* will now be strengthened for the day ahead.

As heart meridian time approaches (11 A.M.–1.00 P.M.), ensure that you have set aside time to nourish baby *yin* by taking a rest, before or after lunch.

As the afternoon passes, the *yang qi* is waning while the *yin qi* is rising (kidney meridian time 5.00 P.M.–7.00 P.M.). Around sunset, therefore, make sure you avoid physical exercise, especially such things as jogging or going to the gym. Instead, slow down, relax and enjoy being quiet, mentally and physically. This will encourage your *yin qi* to grow strong and bring you a calm and refreshing night's sleep.

Once the wheel is turning, you will begin to benefit from the workings of all the meridians, for these make up the other spokes of the wheel and help it to revolve strongly, smoothly, and silently. Remember, too, that in accordance with the cosmos as a hologram, the movement of the wheel signifies not only night and day, but the whole year, baby *yang* time being the winter solstice, sunrise the spring equinox, baby *yin* the summer solstice, and sunset the autumn equinox.

This is *where* to begin. As to *how* to begin, remember to relax! Strain leads only to pain. By relaxing, we harness the power drive of the body.

Some patients turn to meditation in their desire for better health, while others practice meditation for spiritual reasons. Yet without a proper understanding of the body-mind connection, progress is all too often blocked as body syndromes arise, calling for attention but rarely heeded.

The *Dao* is lived in the here-and-now. It teaches us to become aware that although on the surface things appear to be separate, deep down all is flowing as one. This is the way of understanding in the East. So remember that your body is you, just as your spirit is you. Because body and mind are one, the more you learn to listen to your body, the more you open your mind to spirit.

People avoid listening to their bodies if they think they are going to discover something frightening. By using the information system given in this book, you can rest assured that your symptoms are there to help you. Accordingly, the truth is not to be feared, but welcomed.

Now that you understand how *qi* works for you, explore the pages of this book again. Savor the profound wisdom of the *Dao* and benefit from the heritage of five thousand years. Becoming your own physician takes careful study. Be patient with yourself, for you are learning from the great sages of the past, and the book speaks with all the knowledge and wisdom of their authority. We, the authors, applaud you as you take the opportunity to discover how to harness that most precious gift of nature, your *qi*.

Readers interested in finding out more about *qigong* can order the audio compact disk *Point Zero: Practice* Qigong *with Dr. Guo*, with music by Liu Sola, from the Also Productions Inc. Web site at www.alsoproductions.com.

Index

Page numbers in *italics* refer to illustrations.

abdominal breathing, 97, 99–103, *101*
accidents and clumsiness, 42, 43, 63–64, 84, 147–148
acupressure, 60, 62
acupuncture, xvi, 4–5, 17, 57, 62
adenosine monophosphate (AMP), 73–74
aging. *See* longevity
air baths, 116–117, *117*
airplane travel, 146–147
aiye (Artemesia argyi), 34
alcohol: detoxifying the effects of, 111, 112, 138; life span and drunkenness, 95; overeating and, 126–127; proper and improper use of, 136–138; sex and, 142–143; sleep and, 10, 152; use in winter, 106; use while traveling, 146–147
AMP (adenosine monophosphate), 73–74
anger, 76–77
anions, 110
antibiotics, 49, 51
Artemesia argyi, 34
arthritis, 44, 53

asthma, 59–61
aura, 128
automobile travel, 147
autumn, 105–106, 135. *See also* seasons

baby *yang*, 14, 21–23, 152, 160
baby *yin*, 14, 19–20, 152, 160
back problems, 23, 53–56
balance: assessing, 83–87; *dantian*, 30; nutrition and diet, 129; *yin* and *yang*, 11–14, 24–26, 79–80, 93–96, 139–142
bathing, 114–119; after childbirth, 45; after travel, 147; evening, 115–116, 152–153; morning, 97, 114; soaking the feet, 26, 54, 106, 115, 147, 153; winter, 106
beds and bedrooms, 153
belching, 130
benzene molecule, *38*, 38–39
bioelectrical aura, 128
biophotons, 74
biorhythms: and holidays, 64–66; of nature, xv–xvi, 10, 70, 93, 104–106; and travel, 146–147; of *yin* and *yang*, 93–96

bladder meridian, 54–55, *55*
blocked *qi*, 40, *40*, 45–47
blood, 26, 50, 114, 115, 122, 125–126
body functions, normal, 130–131
body/mind relationship, 69–78, 79–80
body-*qi*, 50–51, 64, 75, 105, 114–116, 127, 141–142
body reactions, 81–83. *See also* information-*qi*
brain-wave patterns (EEG), 72
breathing, 99–103
bruises and sprains, 147–148
Buddhism, xvi
burglary, 150

caffeine, 10, 39, 115, 152
cancer, 73–74
case studies: asthma, 59–61; back problems, 53–56; blocked *qi* from wearing rings, 45–47; children's sensitivity to mother's *qi*, 61–63; chronic states of poor health, 49–51; emotional stress, 42–43; heavy menstrual periods, 51–52; holiday syndromes, 63–66; joint problems, 52–53; multiple sclerosis, 56–59; myalgic encephalitis, 47–49; thyroid disorder, 43–45
childbirth. *See* pregnancy and childbirth
children: colorful clothes and, 121; flow of *qi* to and from parents, 61–63, 143; importance of crying, 60–61
China, longevity in, 33–35, 139, 155–157
Chinese fleece flower, 133
Chinese wolfberry, 133, 134
chronic fatigue syndrome, 47–49
chronic ill health, 49–51
climate. *See* environment-*qi*
clothing: colors, 120–122; fit, 122; seasonal, 104, 105, 106, 122

clumsiness. *See* accidents and clumsiness
coffee. *See* caffeine
coherency, 69–70, 74
colds, 47–48, 50–51, 134
collaterals, 15
colors, 120–122
cortisol, 73
countryside, beneficial effects of, 110–111
cravings, 127
creativity, 37–39, 104
crisis *(weiji)*, 41, 86–87
crying, 60–61

daily (twenty-four hour) cycle, *13*, 13–14, 17–18, *18*
damp heat, 44
dantian, 27–30, *28*. *See also* lower *dantian*
Dao, xvii, 70, 161
Daodejing (Dao De Ching), xvi
Daoist tradition: great sages of, xvi–xvii; history, xvi; importance of relaxation, 70; rhythm of life, 95; sex, 142, 143
defecation, 131
dehydration, 107
diaphragm, 101
diet. *See* eating well
digestion, 27–28, 58, 124–127, 138
dihuang, 133
ding neng sheng hui, 39
dizziness, 47, 48
dress. *See* clothing

ears, *8*
eating well, 124–129; breakfast, 98, 125; diet and multiple sclerosis, 58; food preparation, 127–128; how to eat, 124–127; and longevity, 156; nutrition, 128–129; spicy foods, 56; what to eat, 105–106, 127–129
Edison, Thomas, 38

emotions: and colors, 120–122; *dantians* and, 29, 30; effects of stress, 42–43, 72–74, 75–76, 85, 156; role in illness, 75–78
energy-*qi*, 36–41, 61
environment-*qi*: of the home, 149–150; internal climate, 5, 10, 25–26; in nature, 24–25; parent/child flow, 61–63, 143; travel and, 145–146; weather and sex, 142
excesses, effects of, 77–78, 142. *See also* emotions
excess *yang*, 57, 126
exercise. *See* physical exercise/activities
extrasensory perception, 15–16, 29, 82
eyes, as holograms of the body, 9

face map, 7
feet: maps of the soles, 7; nourishing kidney *qi* by keeping warm, 26, 44, 54, 106, *115*, 122–123, 147, 153
fengshui, xvi, xvii, 150
fingers. *See* hands and fingers
fire, 44
five tastes, 129
foods. *See* eating well
forest baths, 119

gallbladder meridian, 21–23, *22*, 56, 77
galvanic skin response, 72–73
Ge Hong, xvii
ginger, 134
ginseng, 132
gouqizi, 133, 134
green tea, 112, 113, 138

hair washing, 115–116
Haiyu, 34
hands and fingers: importance of circulation to, 45, 47; palm maps, 6
headaches, 44, 64, 65

head and upper body, keeping cool, 26, 44, 122–123
health, assessing state of, 49, 83–87
healthy *qi*, 50
heart: and colors red and pink, 121; emotions and, 76, 77; taste associated with, 129
heart meridian, 18–21, *19*, 47
heart *qi*, 55, 116, 140
Heaven Spring water, 112
heshouwu, 133
holiday syndromes, 63–66. *See also* traveling
holograms, 4–9, 54
homes, choosing and furnishing, 149–159, 153
huo, 107, *108*

I Ching (Yijing), xvi, 149
immune system, 50–51, 73–74
information-*qi*: described, 37; in healthy person, 37–39, 83–84; paying attention to, 66, 83; system failure, 86–87, 124; warnings, 39–41, 80–83, 84–85
injuries, 147–148

jet lag, 146–147
jing, 27, 139
joint problems, 44, 52–53

Kekule, Friedrich, 38–39
kidney, 129
kidney meridian, 48, *54*, 57, 152
kidney *qi*: and back problems, 53–54, 56, 57; and the color black, 121; excess fear and, 77; lung problems and, 61; nourishing with warm feet, 54, 106, *115*, 147
Kirlian photography, 128

Laozi (Lao Tsu), xvi
lifestyle, overactive, 42–43, 44–45, 57
Li Shizhen, 136

little *yin*, 13
liuwei dihuang wan, 133–134
liver, 129, 153–154
liver meridian, 153
liver *qi*, 77, 121, 140
longevity, 33–35, 72, 139, 155–157
lower *dantian*, 27–29, 30; and
    asthma, 61; and breathing, 101–
    102, 112; and pregnancy, 143;
    sea of *qi*, 42, 44, 48, 57
lung *qi*, 55, 121, 135, 140
lungs, 58, 77, 100, 129. *See also*
    breathing

mantras, 146, 150
medicated wine, 137
medicinal plants, 132–135
meditation, 153, 160
ME (myalgic encephalitis), 47–49
menstrual periods, 51–52, 139, 143
mental activity: and digestion, 125–
    126; oxygen use during, 100–
    101, 146; and sleep, 152
meridians, 15–18; and the dia-
    phragm, 101; and excessive emo-
    tions, 77; in the fingers, 47; in
    fruit, 128, *129*. *See also specific
    meridians*
metabolic rate, 72, 146–147
midday rest, 10, 13–14, 19–20, 52–
    53, 126
middle *dantian*, 27, 29
mind/body relationship, 69–78, 79–
    80
moon baths, 118–119
morning dew, 111–112
morning routines, 97–98
moxibustion, xvi, 34
multiple sclerosis (MS), 56–59
myalgic encephalitis (ME), 47–49

nature: beneficial effects of trees
    and water, 110–111; biorhythms
    of, 10, 70, 93, 104–106; flow of
    qi in, 16–18, 24–25

nourishing *qi* with warm feet, 26,
    44, 54, 106, *115*, 122–123, 147,
    153
numbers, cardinal, 122

overactive lifestyle, 42–43, 44–45,
    57
overeating and obesity, 95, 124,
    126–127
oxygen consumption, 72, 100–101,
    146–147

painkillers, 40, 49
palm maps, 6
paranormal phenomena, 16, 29, 82
passing wind, 130
pathogenic *qi*: and bathing, 114,
    115; and emotions, 75–76; in the
    home, 149; immune response to,
    50; ridding the body of, 130–
    131; and sweating, 94, 123
physical exercise/activities: after
    eating, 127; evening, 94, 152; and
    longevity, 156; moderation, 95;
    morning, 97; multiple sclerosis
    and, 59; seasonal, 104, 105, 106
physiological responses to stress,
    72–74
pineal gland, 29
plants, medicinal, 132–135
Popp, Fritz, 74
positive reaction, 54, 62
pregnancy and childbirth, 45, 61–
    63, 143, 154

qi: described, 4–5; flow of, 16–18,
    24–26, 40, *40*; functions of, 36–
    41; nourishing with warm feet,
    26, 44, 54, 106, 115, *115*, 122–
    123, 147, 153; sex and, 140. *See
    also* body-*qi*; energy-*qi*; environ-
    ment-*qi*; information-*qi*; patho-
    genic *qi*; sea of *qi*; *yang qi*; *yin qi*;
    specific organs
qi deficiency: assessing levels of, 83–

87; and blood deficiency, 50; sex and, 142; signals of, 39–41, 48, 81

qigong, xvi, xvii, 15; breathing techniques, 99–100; extrasensory perception of practitioners, 15–16, 39; numerical, 122; physiological responses of practitioners, 72–74; saliva and, 108; sex and, 140–141, 144; trees and, 119

radio and television, 10, 98, 125, 127, 152
rainwater, 112
recreation, 156
red dates, 135
relaxation, 70, 160; deep state of, 37–39, 71–74; holidays and, 63–66; protecting *qi*, 88–89
REM (rapid eye movements) sleep, 151–152
rest: following childbirth, 44–45; midday, 10, 13–14, 19–20, 52–53, 126; role in protecting *qi*, 51, 88–89. *See also* relaxation; sleep
rhythms. *See* biorhythms
rings, and obstructed flow of *qi*, 45

saliva, 108, 126, 140
saunas, 116
Schumann Resonance, 72
sea of *qi*, 42–43, 44, 48, 57
seasons, 17, 65, 93, *94*, 104–106, 134–135
seawater, 112
sensitive people, 87, 89
sex, 53, 139–144
shaoyin (little *yin*), 13. *See also* baby *yin*
shen qi, 141
signals, body. *See* information-*qi*
skin, 72–73, 114
sleep, 10, 14, 89, 95, 151–154. *See also* midday rest
small intestine meridian, *46*, 47
smoking, 103, 156

sneezing, 131
spleen, 129
spleen *qi*, 48, 77, 135, 140
sprains and bruises, 147–148
spring, 104–105. *See also* seasons
spring onion and red date tea, 135
stir-frying vegetables, 127–128
stomach, 111, 125
stomach gurgles, 27–28, 102, 130
stomach meridian, 57, 58, *59*
stomach *qi*, 60, 136
stress, effects of, 42–43, 72–74, 75–76, 85, 156
summer, 105, 134–135. *See also* seasons
sun baths, 117–118, *118*
Sun Simiao, xvii, 140–141, 146, 150
sweating, 94, 105, 106, 123

taiji, 11–14, *12*, *13*, 152; with 24-hour cycle of meridians, 17–18, *18*; and the flow of *qi* in nature, 24–26, *25*; of the seasons, 93, *94*; wheel, 160, *160*
taiji (Tai Chi), 71, 97
Tao, 70
TCM. *See* Traditional Chinese Medicine
tea, 112–113, 134–135
television and radio, 10, 98, 125, 127, 152
three worms, 75–76
thyroid disorder, 43–45
tinnitus, 47, 48
tongue: in case study diagnoses, 44, 48, 51, 52, 53, 57, 60, 62; importance in TCM, 5; map of, *9*
Traditional Chinese Medicine (TCM), xvi; alcohol and, 137; approach to sprains and bruises, 147–148; case studies, 42–66; importance of tongue in diagnosis, 4–5; nutrition, 129; principle of the hologram, 4–9; sex, 139–143; uniqueness of each patient, 58

traveling, 145–148
trees, beneficial effects of, 110, 119
turtle breathing, 99–100
twenty-four hour cycle, *13*, 13–14,
    17–18, *18*

universe, 3–4, 11–12. *See also* nature
upper body and head, keeping cool,
    26, 44, 122–123
upper *dantian*, 27, 29, 30
urination, 131
uroboros, *38*, 38–39

vacations, 63–66. *See also* traveling
volcano effect, 44, 123

washing. *See* bathing
water: external sources of, 109–113;
    internal (body water), 107–109
Wei Boyang, xvi–xvii
weiji (crisis), 41, 86–87
wine. *See* alcohol
wine bottle analogy, 84–87
winter, 65, 106. *See also* seasons
worms, three, 75–76

Xie Huanzhang, 74
x-ray vision, 15–16
xunlaowan, 133

yang: biorhythms of, 93–94, 104–
    105; healthy balance, 83–87; in
    nature, 24–26; and sex, 139–142;
    and the *Taiji*, 11–14. *See also*
    baby *yang*

yang deficiency, 20–21, 23, 51
yang meridians, 17, *17*
yang qi: afternoon activities and, 94,
    116; digestion and, 124, 125–
    126; midday rest and, 21, 22–23;
    pathogenic *qi* and, 50, 94; sea-
    sonal changes, 104–106; sex and,
    139; water temperature and,
    111, 114–115
yawning, 131
*The Yellow Emperor's Canon of Med-
    icine*, xvi, 56, 104, 129
Yijing (I Ching), xvi, 149
yin: biorhythms of, 93–96, 105–
    106; healthy balance, 83–87; in
    nature, 24–26; and sex, 139–142;
    and the *Taiji*, 11–14. *See also*
    baby *yin*
yin deficiency: alcohol consumption,
    137; asthma, 60; back problems,
    53, 56; heart meridian, 20; morn-
    ing dew and moist air and, 111–
    112; multiple sclerosis, 57; signs
    of, 51–52, 52–53, 94–95; vaca-
    tions and, 64–65
yin meridians, 17, *17*
yin qi: digestion and, 124; moon and
    forest baths, 118–119; from
    morning dew and moist air, 111–
    112; nourishing, 94–95, 152; sea-
    sonal changes, 104–106; sex and,
    139

Zhang Changlin, 74

About the Authors

BISONG GUO was born in China and studied Western medicine at Fuzhou Medical School before specializing in Traditional Chinese Medicine. She later joined the staff of the Chinese Academy of Traditional Chinese Medicine in Beijing. For more than twenty-five years she has intensively practiced *qigong*, studying with Buddhist *qigong* masters and Daoist monks in remote mountainous regions of China. In 1989 she moved to England and established a TCM practice in Newcastle-upon-Tyne, where over ten years she treated more than five thousand patients. She has collaborated on research projects in Germany and now travels widely overseas conducting seminars and workshops. Dr. Guo continues to teach *qigong* in the United Kingdom, continental Europe, and the United States.

ANDREW POWELL graduated from Cambridge University with distinction in medicine and, after further studies in general medicine and psychiatry, specialized in psychotherapy at the Maudsley Hospital, London. He was Consultant and Senior Lecturer at St. George's Hospital, London, for eleven years before moving to Oxford, where he continued to work in the National Health Service until 2000. He has a special interest in the influence of spiritual dynamics on physical and psychological well-being and in the study of Eastern approaches to consciousness. Dr. Powell is an Associate of the College of Healing and Founder Chairman of the Spirituality and Psychiatry Special Interest Group of the Royal College of Psychiatrists, United Kingdom.